TECHNICAL REPORT

T0195491

Tests to Evaluate Public Health Disease Reporting Systems in Local Public Health Agencies

David J. Dausey, Nicole Lurie, Alexis Diamond,
Barbara Meade, Roger C. Molander, Karen Ricci,
Michael A. Stoto, Jeffrey Wasserman

Prepared for the U.S. Department of Health and Human Services

RAND

Center for Domestic and
International Health Security

A RAND HEALTH PROGRAM

The research described in this report was carried out under the auspices of the RAND Center for Domestic and International Health Security, a program within RAND Health, and was sponsored by the U.S. Department of Health and Human Services.

ISBN 0-8330-3827-3

The RAND Corporation is a nonprofit research organization providing objective analysis and effective solutions that address the challenges facing the public and private sectors around the world. RAND's publications do not necessarily reflect the opinions of its research clients and sponsors.

RAND® is a registered trademark.

Published 2005 by the RAND Corporation
1776 Main Street, P.O. Box 2138, Santa Monica, CA 90407-2138
1200 South Hayes Street, Arlington, VA 22202-5050
201 North Craig Street, Suite 202, Pittsburgh, PA 15213-1516
RAND URL: http://www.rand.org/
To order RAND documents or to obtain additional information, contact
Distribution Services: Telephone: (310) 451-7002;
Fax: (310) 451-6915; Email: order@rand.org

Preface

The importance of public health disease reporting systems cannot be overstated in an age of increasing globalization, when localized naturally occurring outbreaks can have a global reach and the threat of bioterrorism is very real. Despite the importance of these systems, few standardized tools have been developed to help public health agencies evaluate their effectiveness.

This operations manual aims to fill this gap by providing public health agencies with a set of standardized proficiency tests to aid in the development of regular and consistent strategies for testing public health disease reporting systems. The tests are intended to evaluate the ability to receive and respond to case reports 24 hours a day, 7 days a week. We refined these tests by beta-testing them at 20 metropolitan area local public health agencies across the country over the course of 10 months.

The contents of this manual will be of interest to public health professionals at the state and local level that are responsible for ensuring that their public health disease reporting systems are functioning appropriately.

This work was supported by the U.S. Department of Health and Human Services under Contract No. 282-00-0005, for which Dr. William Raub, Principal Deputy Assistant Secretary for Public Health Emergency Preparedness, is the project officer. The research was produced within RAND Health's Center for Domestic and International Health Security. RAND Health is a division of the RAND Corporation.

Table of Contents

Table of Figures

Table of Tables

Acknowledgements

This manual is one part of a larger project being conducted by the RAND Corporation, with funding from the U.S. Department of Health and Human Services, to examine exemplary public health practices, learn from public health experiences, and develop exercises to improve public health preparedness. We would like to acknowledge and thank the entire RAND team on this project for their efforts, many of which helped shape our thinking and approach to this work.

Developing this operations manual involved the participation of dozens of public health professionals from 20 metropolitan area local public health agencies across the country. We are deeply grateful for their willingness to participate in the tests and to provide us with constructive feedback while we beta-tested the manual. We would like especially to thank Dr. Raoult Ratard, State Epidemiologist at the Louisiana Office of Public Health, and Dr. Michael Seid at the RAND Corporation for their in-depth reviews.

We would also like to acknowledge the assistance and guidance of Dr. William Raub, Principal Deputy Assistant Secretary for Public Health Emergency Preparedness, and Ms. Lara Lamprecht, Program Analyst, of the Office of the Assistant Secretary for Public Health Emergency Preparedness at the U.S. Department of Health and Human Services. Their commitment to developing tools and resources to help public health agencies improve the country's public health preparedness was the driving force behind this work.

Chapter 1.
Introduction

This manual is designed to aid in the development of *proficiency tests*[1] intended to evaluate the ability of public health disease reporting systems at *local public health agencies* (LPHA) to receive and respond to *case reports* 24 hours a day, 7 days a week (24/7). Its four primary objectives are to:
- Serve as a guidebook for planning a test
- Serve as a training and reference manual for individuals conducting a test
- Provide tools and templates necessary to conduct the tests
- Provide benchmarks to evaluate testing performance.

The goal of these tests is to assess whether a LPHA has sufficient proficiency to respond to public health disease reports as outlined by the Centers for Disease Control and Prevention (CDC, 1988, 2001, 2003). It is intended that these tests be used over time to regularly monitor and improve performance of public health disease reporting systems.

The manual outlines four phases for planning and conducting a test:
- Planning a test—identifying a testing agency, choosing an appropriate test, selecting staff, materials required to conduct tests, and developing call schedules
- Training to conduct a test—trainer responsibilities, preparing for a test, learning to debrief, and practice and observation
- Conducting a test—initiating a call, reaching an action officer, and debriefing
- Assessing test performance—creating an after-action report and evaluation benchmarks

Figure 1.1 highlights how these phases relate to the manual's objectives.

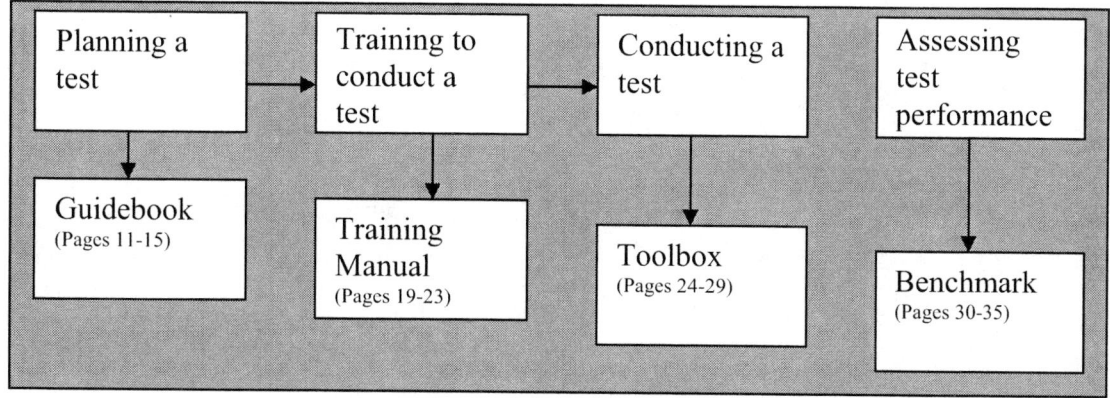

Figure 1.1 Structure of Operations Manual

---

[1] Appendix A contains definitions for all terms in the manual that appear in italics.

SIGNIFICANCE

Public health disease reporting systems are one of the first lines of defense in identifying a public health emergency (Jajosky and Groseclose, 2004). Since September 11, 2001 and the subsequent anthrax attacks, strengthening the public health infrastructure, including disease reporting systems, has been a national priority (Henderson, 2003). The importance of responsive, well-coordinated reporting systems – that work 24/7– cannot be overstated. The ultimate goal of these systems is the early detection of outbreaks before they have a chance to spread widely through the population (Buehler et. al, 2004). Testing of 24/7 responsiveness at least annually is one of the CDC's Performance Criteria, and is a key responsibility of every LPHA (CDC, 2003).

One of the best ways to find out if reporting systems are functioning properly is to test them. Despite the importance of such tests, few standardized testing tools have been developed. This manual aims to fill this gap by providing a set of standardized proficiency tests to aid in the development of regular and consistent strategies for testing and evaluating public health disease reporting systems.

INTENDED AUDIENCE

This manual is intended for the leadership of LPHAs (e.g., public health directors and *bioterrorism coordinators*) who are responsible for ensuring that that their public health agency is capable of responding to case reports in a timely and efficient manner. This manual is not intended public health professionals directly involved in responding to case reports—these individuals are part of the system to be tested.

ROADMAP

The rest of this manual is divided into six chapters. Chapter 2 introduces testing strategies for evaluating public health disease reporting systems. It begins by discussing the basic concepts and terminology for public health disease reporting systems. It then outlines strategies for testing these systems and discusses a variety of different testing formats.

Chapters 3 through 6 discuss the four phases for developing and conducting a test. The final chapter of the manual describes strategies for public health professionals to use to develop regular, formal, standardized systems for testing their public health disease reporting systems.

Chapter 2.
Testing Public Health Disease Reporting Systems

Public health disease reporting systems are systems developed by public health agencies to receive and respond to cases reported to them by healthcare professionals that have public health significance. The CDC recommends telephone calls as the preferred method for public health agencies to receive case reports of an urgent nature (CDC, 2003). These *concerning cases* or urgent cases represent potential public health threats that need to be responded to immediately. Calls regarding concerning cases can come from a variety of places and individuals, including infectious disease practitioners at local hospitals, doctors in private practice, and nurses working at nursing homes. The public health agency must respond to concerning case reports in a timely and appropriate way. A timely response means that a public health professional responds to the call within 30 minutes. Appropriate means that there is an adequate strategy for triaging calls and that staff with requisite levels of training and clinical knowledge are available to respond. Figure 2.1 highlights the general processes involved in public health disease reporting systems.

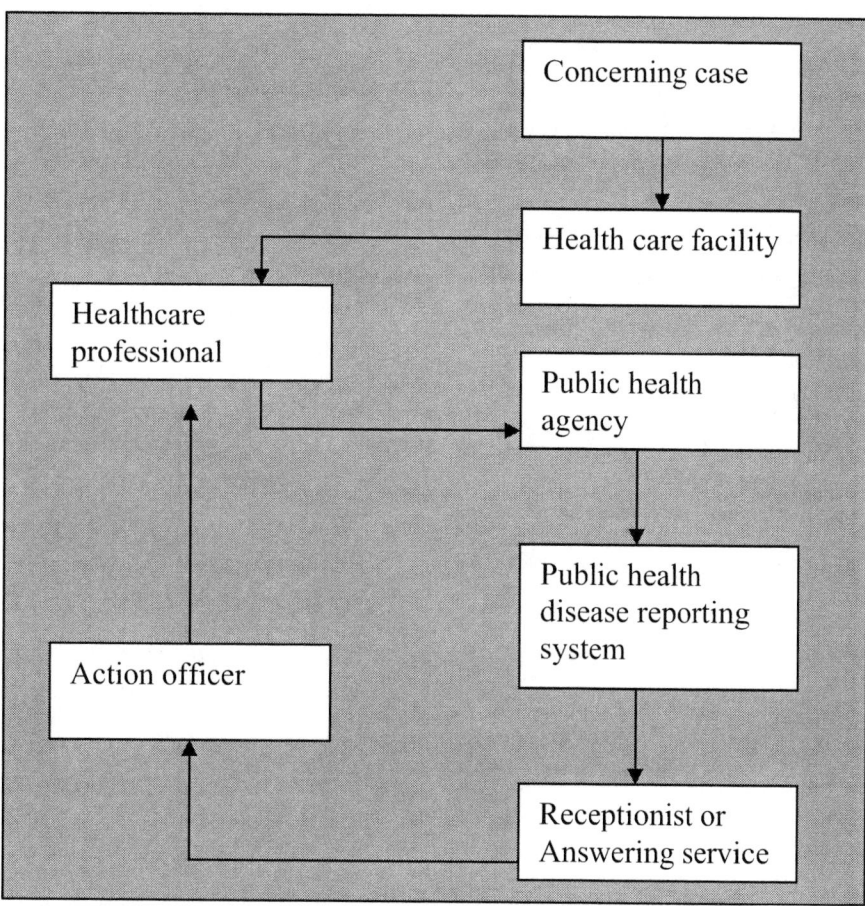

Figure 2.1 General Processes Involved in Public Health Disease Reporting Systems

GENERAL TESTING FORMAT

Several different testing strategies to evaluate public health disease reporting systems are discussed in this manual. All of the strategies share three common elements:

- Initiating a call
- Reaching an action officer
  - Warm transfer
  - Callback
- Debriefing

"Initiating a call" means that the caller (the person conducting the test) phones a public health agency directly and, using a lead-in, asks to speak with an appropriate action officer. The *lead-in* is the message intended to move a call from a reception desk, switchboard, or answering service to an action officer.

An *action officer* is the public health professional at the public health agency responsible for responding to public health emergencies during the time of a call. Action officers can be public health directors, epidemiologists, bioterrorism coordinators, doctors, nurses, etc. "Reaching an action officer" may involve a warm transfer or a callback.

A *warm transfer* is when the caller is immediately transferred to an action officer. However, not every call will result in immediate contact with an appropriate action officer. The caller may be required to leave a message with a telephone number for the action officer to call as soon as he or she receives the message. A *callback* occurs when an action officer returns the call. Once the caller reaches a respondent, it is necessary to verify that the person returning the call is actually an appropriate action officer. All calls end with a "debriefing."

Debriefing is when the caller discusses the call with the action officer, answers any questions the action officer may have, and ensures that the action officer fully understands that the call is only a test and requires no further action. Debriefing procedures are discussed in more detail later in this chapter.

ADVANCED NOTIFICATION AND THE USE OF DISGUISE

Public health disease reporting systems should be tested in an environment that is as realistic as possible. Two features have the greatest influence over the test's realism: advance notification and the use of a disguise. A *disguise* refers to the use of role-playing by the caller to enhance the realism of a test. A typical disguise involves a caller pretending to be a healthcare professional calling a public health agency about a concerning case.

Figure 2.2 highlights these testing aspects on a realism continuum. Preplanned announced tests that do not involve a disguise are the least realistic; completely unannounced tests that involve using a disguise are the most realistic. Chapter 3 will help you select the level of test that is right for your agency. The test templates described in this manual include preplanned announced tests, announced but unscheduled tests, and completely unannounced tests. Preplanned announced tests are tests in which public health staff are told that there will be a test of their public health disease reporting system during a defined time period (e.g., the month of November). Announced but unscheduled tests are tests in which public health staff are told that their public health agency's disease reporting system will be evaluated some time in the future. The test could take place six months—or one day—after the announcement. Completely unannounced tests are tests in which public health staff receives no notification of the test at all.

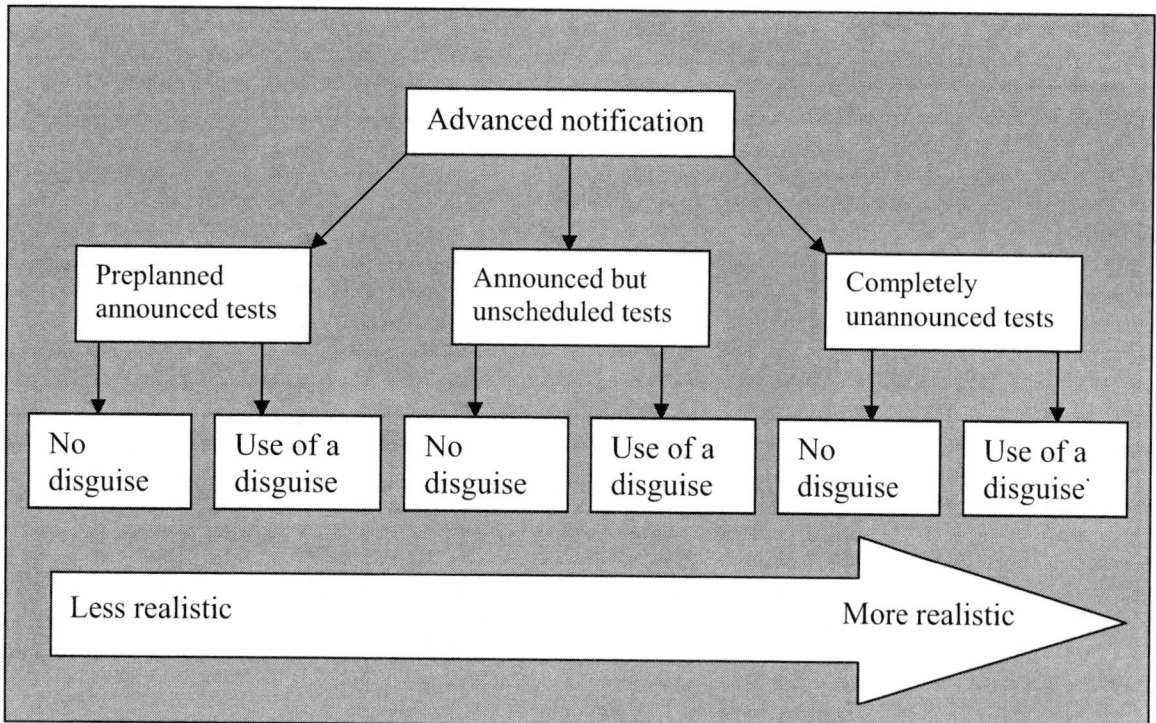

Figure 2.2 Continuum of Realism

The tests described in this manual can be used with or without disguise. However, test planners should keep in mind that the use of disguise greatly enhances the realism of a test. There are several ways in which disguise can be used; however, the most basic is during call initiation. An example of a test with no disguise is when the caller says during call initiation: "This is a test. Please provide a callback by an appropriate action officer as soon as possible." An example of a test with disguise is when the caller says during call initiation: "This is Doctor Smith from Community Hospital, and I have a concerning case involving an infectious disease that I would like to talk to someone about." The response to the test that does not involve a disguise is likely to be different than a response to a more realistic test involving a disguise.

Even announced tests can involve a disguise that can increase the realism of the test. If the test involves a disguise, every effort should be made to sustain the disguise for the entire testing period. *Detection* occurs when staff members at a public health agency become aware that their agency is being tested.

Several strategies can be used to avoid detection, including
- Spacing and timing the calls appropriately
- Purchasing a cellular phone to make the calls from a phone number local to the LPHA called
- Using a disguise during call initiation
- Asking respondents who have responded to a call not to discuss the call with their co-workers.

AVOIDING FALSE ALARMS

While the use of disguises greatly increases a test's realism, there is an accompanying danger: false alarms (incidents in which a false report triggers a public health response). To avoid this possibility, callers must be well trained in "debriefing" and other call management issues. The key to avoiding a false alarm is that after reaching an action officer callers should never hang up the phone until the action officer is properly debriefed. See Chapter 5 for more details on debriefing and strategies to avoid false alarms.

TESTING LEVELS

There are four different *testing levels* described in this manual. Each is progressively more challenging. Levels 1, 2, and 3 can involve using a disguise or may be conducted without a disguise.[2] Level 4 (which is the most challenging) involves the use of a disguise. Each progressive testing level has operational goals that build upon the goals of the previous Level. Table 2.1 highlights the capabilities each level is designed to test. When choosing among testing levels, the operational goals of the testing level should be matched with the operational goals of the public health agency. For example, to test timeliness only, choose a Level 1 test. To test timeliness plus procedural knowledge, choose Level 2. To test timeliness and procedural knowledge plus content knowledge, choose Level 3. To test all four capabilities (timeliness, procedural knowledge, content knowledge, and stress management skills), choose Level 4.

Level 1 tests are the most basic. The caller is responsible for recording the answers to eight questions related to the timeliness of response:
- Was the call answered within 5 rings? (yes/no)
- How long was the wait time on hold? (in minutes)
- Was the call transferred in 5 rings? (yes/no)
- Did the call involve a warm transfer or a callback? (yes/no)
- Was the call a *dead end*? (yes/no)
- Did an appropriate action officer respond on first warm transfer or callback? (yes/no)

---

[2] Techniques for conducting the actual tests and for using disguise are only introduced here. They are described in greater detail in Chapters 4 and 5.

- How long was the wait for the callback? (in minutes)
- Was the callback received in 30 minutes or less? (yes/no)

Level 1 tests begin when the caller initiates a call to a public health agency that requires contact with an action officer. The test ends when the caller reaches an appropriate action officer. A disguise can be used in Level 1 tests during call initiation to increase the realism of the test. As soon as the action officer responds to the call, the caller should immediately debrief the action officer and explain that the call is a test and that no further action is required. Public health agencies are organized in different ways, so determining if the respondent is an appropriate action officer may require caller probes (e.g., "Are you the appropriate person to handle a case report?" "What is your title?" etc.). Action officer titles should suggest whether they have enough clinical knowledge to respond to a case report.

For example, doctors, nurses, and epidemiologists would have such knowledge, while an entomologist or a student intern at the public health agency probably would not. The caller must use his or her own judgment to determine whether the respondent is an appropriate action officer. If an inappropriate respondent responds to the call, the caller should ask that respondent to notify an appropriate action officer and request another callback.

Table 2.1 Operational Goals Tested in Each Testing Level

Goal	Level 1	Level 2	Level 3	Level 4
Speed of Response From call initiation to action officer's initial response	●	●	●	●
Procedural Knowledge Action officer understands procedures and triage system		●	●	●
Content Knowledge Action officer is familiar with basic epidemiology and sequelae of agent/disease in case report			●	●
Stress Management Action officer is capable of balanced understanding and response to an urgent case under stressful circumstances				●

Level 2 tests assess both the timeliness of the response (the same as Level 1) and the responder's procedural knowledge. Initiating the call and the debriefing procedure for Level 2 tests is the same as Level 1. The procedure after receiving a callback, however, is slightly different. After reaching an appropriate action officer and explaining that the call is a test, the caller asks the action officer questions about how calls are triaged at his or her public health agency and questions regarding the action officer's procedural knowledge about responding to calls.

The caller will note answers to the following questions:
- Did the action officer know and understand their public health agency's triage protocol for concerning case reports?
- Was the action officer aware of their public health agency's ability to record calls for quality assurance?
- Did the action officer know anything about the surge capacity of their public health disease reporting system?
- Did the action officer know whether or not he or she could initiate a three-way call for concerning case reports?
- Was the action officer aware of a backup action officer who was available during the time of the call?

Level 3 tests assess timeliness of the response and procedural knowledge (the same as Level 2) and the respondent's content knowledge. Level 3 procedures for initiating the call and the debriefing tests are the same as for Level 2. However, after reaching an appropriate action officer and explaining that the call is a test, Level 3 tests assess content knowledge in addition to procedural knowledge.

Content knowledge is tested by reading a brief description of a concerning case report and asking the action officer to identify appropriate next steps. The caller will note answers to the following questions:
- Was the action officer able to determine the disease being discussed in the case report without being told?
- Did the action officer know what to tell the caller to do next?
- Did the action officer discuss personal protective equipment with the caller without first being probed?
- Did the action officer ask for more case details after hearing case report?

If the action officer is unable to respond to the case report, the caller should request that the action officer contact a more informed individual and have that person contact the caller as soon as possible. The test does not end until the caller reaches an action officer who is able to respond to the case report.

Adequate responses to the case report involve the action officer describing what he or she would do next from the public health agency's perspective as well as recommending to the caller what next steps the caller should take to care for the case (e.g., using personal protective equipment, placing the case in an isolation room, limiting the number of staff who come into contact with the case).

Level 4 tests are the most challenging. They are completely unannounced and require callers to use a disguise. Callers initiate calls to public health agencies by reporting a concerning case that requires a response from an action officer. When the action officer responds to the call, the caller, instead of immediately debriefing the officer, pretends to be a healthcare worker, describes a concerning case, and asks what to do next. After the action officer details his/her response, the caller debriefs the action officer. It is critical that the caller never hang up with an action officer without first telling the officer that the call is a test.

Content knowledge is assessed by reading a brief description of a concerning case report and asking the action officer what should be done next. The caller will note answers to the following questions:
- Was the action officer able to determine the disease being discussed in the case report without being told?
- Did the action officer know what to tell the caller to do next?
- Did the action officer discuss personal protective equipment with the caller without first being probed?
- Did the action officer ask for more case details after hearing the case report?

DEBRIEFING PROCEDURES

Every person who comes into contact with a caller should be properly debriefed (e.g., receptionists, action officers, etc.). This includes respondents to Level 1 calls and respondents to calls that do not involve using a disguise.

Debriefing for all levels involves:
- Clarification that the call is a test that requires no further action
- General information about the tests and testing procedures
- Contact information for the testing supervisor or coordinator
- Questions for respondents.

Debriefing occurs immediately after receiving a callback from an action officer for all calls except Level 4 calls. For Level 4 calls, the caller first presents the action officer with a concerning case report and asks what steps and procedures should be taken next. Debriefing occurs after the action officer answers.

No callback should ever be terminated or placed on hold unless the respondent is first debriefed. If a call is accidentally disconnected during a callback, the caller should immediately try to contact the action officer again and should continue to do so until contact is resumed and the debriefing is complete.

All debriefings begin by telling the respondent that the call is a test that requires no further action. This is most important for calls that involve a disguise and especially for Level 4 calls. However, debriefing is important even for calls that do not involve using a disguise to avoid confusion about the purpose of the call.

Respondents should then be told that the test is part of ongoing public health agency efforts to ensure that the public health disease reporting system at the public health agency is functioning properly. The caller should tell the respondent the name of the individual at the public health agency that authorized the test.

During the debriefing, callers should ask respondents if they have any questions about the call they received. Questions a caller cannot answer should be directed to the testing coordinator.

Some respondents may be upset or react defensively to test calls. Callers should attempt to diffuse these situations by explaining to respondents that the tests are not an evaluation of individuals but instead an evaluation of systems and that there are many places in the response system that can break down. Callers should highlight the importance of testing public health disease reporting systems to identify problems that may exist with these systems and to develop strategies to overcome these problems. Respondents who are not satisfied with these responses should be referred to the testing coordinator. Debriefings for calls that involve using a disguise should end by asking the respondent not to talk to others in their agency about the call. Debriefing templates are included in Appendix E.

Chapter 3.
Planning a Test

A successful test is the result of good planning. A number of factors should be considered before testing including the unique characteristics of the public health agency to be tested (e.g., size of agency, number of affiliated hospitals, urban versus rural, etc.), choosing an appropriate test (e.g., level of difficulty, number of calls, using a disguise, etc.), and the staffing needs of the test. This chapter describes how to successfully plan a test. Figure 3.1 highlights the framework for these activities.

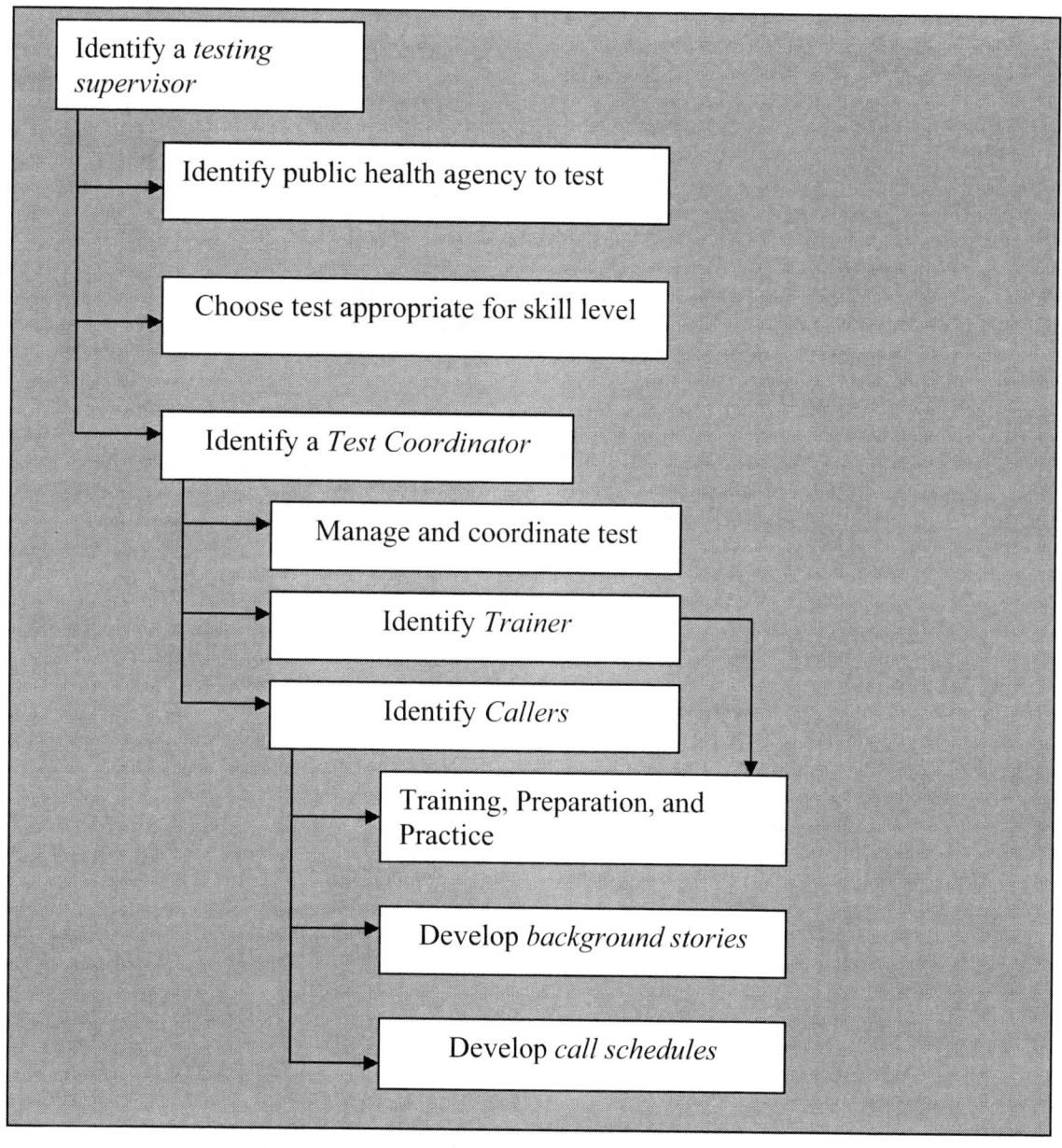

Figure 3.1 Framework for Planning a Test

STAFFING AND MATERIALS

The categories of staff needed to develop and conduct a test include:
- Supervisor
- Testing coordinator (may be the same person as supervisor)
- Trainer(s) (may be the same person as testing coordinator)[3]
- Caller(s).

The *supervisor* is the individual with the authority to conduct a test. The supervisor provides supervision for the entire testing period. The supervisor may also choose to coordinate the tests or may choose a designee to handle the day-to-day coordination of testing activities. The *testing coordinator* is in charge of planning and coordinating tests, ensuring staff is properly trained, and answering any questions both callers or respondents might have about the exercises. The *trainer* is responsible for planning, coordinating, and running training sessions for new callers. The *callers* are responsible for placing the calls and recording the responses.

The total number of staff and total staff time required to conduct a test depends on four factors:
- Total number of calls to be conducted
- The timeframe in which the calls are to be conducted
- Total number of public health agencies being tested
- Level of test chosen.

The total number of callers necessarily depends on the factors mentioned above. Unless multiple public health agencies are being tested by one testing agency, one to three callers working part time (5–10 hours a week) are all that are typically necessary to conduct a test. In order to truly test a public health agency's ability to respond to case reports 24/7/365 it may be necessary to pay callers overtime to make calls after hours on weekdays or during weekends. As the number of calls desired increases and the timeframe in which the calls are to be conducted decreases, the total number of staff needed to conduct the calls increases.

Four different tests are possible (described in detail later in this chapter). However, you may decide you need only a subset of these tests. Very few materials are required to conduct a test. Ideally, callers should have access to a computer with software that allows them to track and record their calls (e.g., MS Excel, Access, etc.); however, this can be done without a computer. Callers will also need access to a dedicated telephone line to place their calls. To avoid detection, the testing agency may decide to purchase cellular telephones with phone numbers local to the LPHAs. Cellular telephones offer the advantage that callers can carry them and can use them outside of an office.

The disadvantage to cellular phones is the fact that in some areas and locations they may not work because of limited service regions and barriers that prevent proper

---

[3] The roles and responsibilities of the trainer are discussed in Chapter 4.

transmission of calls (e.g., being inside a large building when placing a call). Therefore, all telephone lines used for callbacks need to have message systems for respondents who call back and are unable to reach the caller. The outgoing message should clearly state that the call was a test, that the person calling should leave a message to confirm the callback, and that no further action is required.

CHOOSING A TESTING AGENCY

The *testing agency* is the agency or organization conducting the test. Testing agencies can include:

- State public health agencies evaluating the performance of LPHAs in their state
- LPHAs self-evaluating their public health disease reporting systems
- LPHAs partnering with other LPHAs to independently evaluate one another
- LPHAs contracting with an outside vendor to conduct the tests for them.

The test templates provided in this manual can be customized to work in any one of these scenarios.

Every public health agency should have a well-developed disease reporting system. However, the reality is that some are still in an early stage of development. Conducting premature tests in these agencies is likely to cause frustration and anger among the staff. Instead, these agencies should be encouraged to develop a more sophisticated case reporting system. Once they develop such a system, the system can be tested to evaluate its proficiency.

To avoid a potential false alarm, it is usually best that at least one high-level leader at the public health agency being tested is aware that a test is occurring. Depending on the relationship between the testing agency and the public health agency to be tested, it may be necessary to obtain the consent of director of that public health agency to participate in a test. Even if it is not necessary, consent is generally advisable.

CHOOSING AN APPROPRIATE TEST

Choosing a test template appropriate for the skill level of a public health agency involves the discernment of the testing supervisor. There are three decisions that must be made before any test can be developed:

- Level of advance notification (preplanned, unscheduled, unannounced)
- Use of a disguise (yes/no)
- Choice of test level (1–4)

Taken together, these options yield 21 different broad test templates as highlighted by Table 3.1. Each of the test templates can be customized to yield an even larger number of potential tests.

Table 3.1 Complete Matrix of Test Templates

Use of a Disguise[4]	Advanced Notification		
	Preplanned	Unscheduled	Unannounced
No	Test Level 1	Test Level 1	Test Level 1
	Test Level 2	Test Level 2	Test Level 2
	Test Level 3	Test Level 3	Test Level 3
Yes	Test Level 1	Test Level 1	Test Level 1
	Test Level 2	Test Level 2	Test Level 2
	Test Level 3	Test Level 3	Test Level 3
	Test Level 4	Test Level 4	Test Level 4

Each of these testing templates can be placed on a continuum of difficulty measured in terms of complexity and intellectual and emotional challenge (Figure 3.2).

For the caller, moving right on the continuum of difficulty requires increasing levels of:
- Understanding of epidemiologic responses
- Familiarity with public health agency-specific response protocols
- Clinical and disease knowledge for placing case reports
- Debriefing complexity
- Stress associated with placing calls

These requirements can largely be met through preparation and practice (as outlined in Chapter 4).

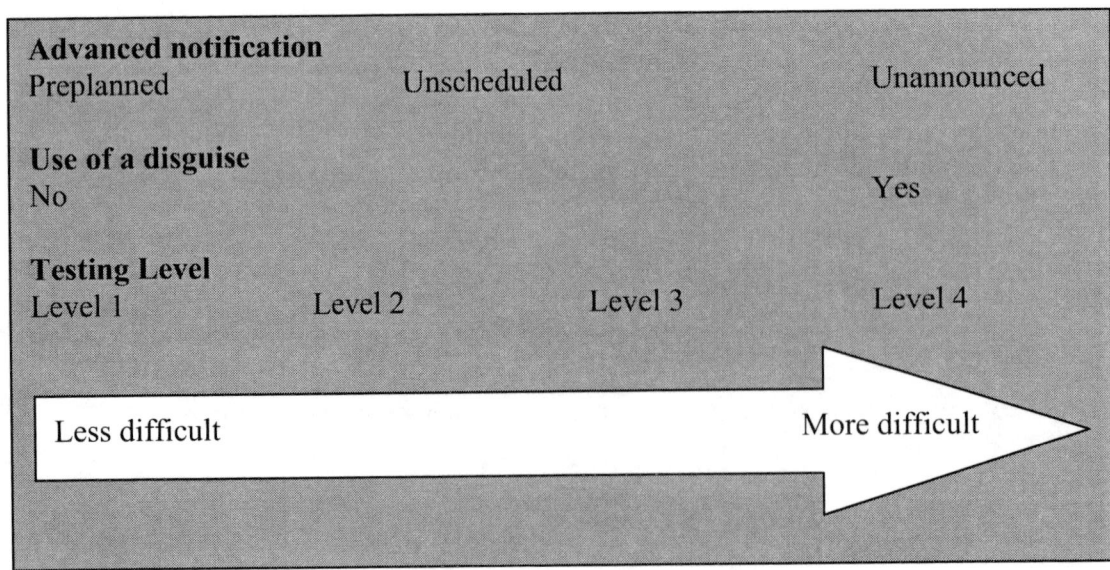

Figure 3.2 Continuum of Testing Templates

---

[4] Level 4 tests cannot be conducted without the use of disguise, which is why they are not included in the row disguise = no.

For the action officer, moving right on the continuum of difficulty requires increasing levels of:

- Procedural knowledge of disease reporting protocols
- Content knowledge of agent / disease epidemiology, clinical characteristics, and sequelae
- Stress associated with the call.

The test chosen should be challenging for the public health agency to be tested but not overwhelming. Public health agencies with new disease reporting systems or protocols or public health agencies with disease reporting systems that do not operate 24/7/365 should be given tests that are less difficult. Public health agencies with established disease reporting systems that have protocols in place for responding to case reports 24/7/365 can be given tests that are more difficult. Furthermore, when choosing a test, the caller's level of experience should also be considered. Callers should have experience with the preceding level before going on to the next level.

The tests developed in this manual have been designed to be part of a regular testing protocol that public health agencies can use over time to continually improve the quality of their case reporting systems. The feedback public health agencies receive after each test can be used to improve their case reporting systems. These systems can then later be retested to evaluate the success of these improvements. As a public health agency's case reporting system improves, the agency should be given tests of increasing difficulty until it is able to successfully handle the most difficult tests. Public health agencies that reach this point should then be regularly tested to ensure that they maintain this level of proficiency over time as staff and leadership at the department changes.

DEVELOPING CALL SCHEDULES AND BACKGROUND STORIES

Calls to participating public health agencies should be planned in advance. A typical test of one public health agency involves 10 calls to a public health agency over the course of 1–2 months. Prior to testing, the testing coordinator should develop a call schedule for each public health agency to be tested that takes into account the total number of calls and timeframe of the calls to be conducted. A *call schedule* is a calendar that identifies the dates and times for calls as well as the callers responsible for placing the calls.

Creating a call schedule is important for three reasons. First, it ensures that enough time is set aside in advance for each call to be conducted. For example, Level 3 and 4 calls, including preparation, can last for as long as 30–60 minutes, not including any time spent waiting for a callback. Consequently, it is important to set aside ample time to properly make, receive, and conduct calls.

Second, call schedules ensure that the participating public health agency receives calls at different times and different days of the week, thus better testing its 24-7 capacity. The work schedule of a targeted public health agency can be broken into weekdays (i.e., Monday through Friday) and weekends. Each of these can be further delineated into morning, lunch, afternoon, and after hours. Calls should be scheduled such that you initiate contact with the participating public health agency at most (if not all) of the various aforementioned times, both during the week and on the weekend.

Third, for calls that involve using a disguise, call schedules can help callers to avoid detection. Calls that involve disguise need to be scheduled such that participating public health agencies remain unaware of the test. Therefore, a public health agency's size and the number of its hospital affiliates are two factors that should be used to determine how best to space the scheduling of phone calls. Smaller public health agencies may need calls spaced further apart to avoid detection while medium and large sized public health agencies may be able to be tested in shorter time frames. The response of most public health agencies can be evaluated with 6–10 calls.

As a rule of thumb:
- Small public health agencies that serve fewer than three hospitals and have fewer than four staff members responding to case reports should receive no more than one call a week.
- Medium to large sized public health agencies that serve three or more hospitals and have five or more staff members responding to case reports can receive two or more calls in one week.

There are a number of different approaches to developing call schedules. One way to ensure calls are distributed across different days and times is to use a "menu approach." Figure 3.3 provides an example of such an approach for a public health agency that is scheduled to receive 10 calls.

The caller responsible for making calls to this public health agency would need to develop a call schedule that adhered to the scheduling guidelines suggested based on the number of weeks of testing. In this example, testing would involve a minimum of five weeks' time (e.g., ten calls, but no more than two calls per week).

In addition to the dates, times, and names of the callers placing the tests, call schedules should also include the telephone number that the caller needs to call to reach the public health agency action officer. This number may be obtained from a variety of sources, including (but not limited to):
- Local telephone directory assistance (CDC recommendation)
- Public health agency web page
- Public health agency instructions for after-hours emergencies.

More than one number may exist. The person developing the call schedule should make sure that the callers test all plausible telephone numbers that the public health agency has listed.

Column A	Column B	Column C	Column D	Column E
5:00am–5:59am	8:00am–8:59am	12:00pm–12:59pm	2:00pm–2:59pm	6:00pm–7:59pm
6:00am–6:59am	9:00am–9:59am	1:00pm–1:59pm	3:00pm–3:59pm	8:00pm–9:59pm
7:00am–7:59am	10:00am–10:59am		4:00pm–4:59pm	10:00pm–11:59pm
	11:00am–11:59am		5:00pm–5:59pm	12:00am–4:59am

For weekdays:
Must choose 1 from Column A (early morning before most regular staff arrives to work)
Must choose 2 from Column B (normal morning working hours)
Must choose 2 from Column C (lunch time when some staff may be away from the office)
Must choose 2 from Column D (normal afternoon working hours)
Must choose 1 from Column E (after hours and late night)

For weekends:
Must choose 1 from column A or E
Must choose 1 from column B, C or D

At least 1 call must be made on each day of the week
No more than 2 calls per week

Figure 3.3 Example of Menu Approach to Scheduling Call Times

The person obtaining the telephone number for the public health agency to be tested should record:
- Single number available for all calls day or night? (yes/no)
- Telephone number available through local directory assistance? (yes/no)
- Single telephone number well publicized? (e.g., same number found in more than one source, such as on the Internet and from directory assistance)? (yes/no)
- Total number of telephone numbers at public health agency related to public health disease reporting.

Appendix F includes a sample data collection form.

Callers should be instructed to record telephone numbers that lead to dead ends. A *dead end* occurs when callers reach the end of an automated telephone recording system and are not given the opportunity to leave a message or are not provided with another telephone number to call in an emergency.

For calls that involve disguise, callers will need a background story for use during call initiation. A *background story* contains four elements:
- Fictitious name of a healthcare professional making the call (e.g., Doctor Smith, Nurse Jones)

17

- Background of healthcare professional (e.g., emergency medicine physician, infection control practitioner, nurse practitioner)
- Name of local healthcare facility where healthcare professional is calling (e.g., name of a local hospital, nursing home)
- Vague case information (e.g., a concerning case involving an infectious disease).

Appropriate background stories should be developed by the caller and the test coordinator. All of this information should be established prior to making the call, and it should be changed (at least marginally) for every call to reduce the likelihood of detection. All of the information needed for a background story can be fictitious except for the name of the local healthcare facility. In order to keep calls that involve disguise as realistic as possible, the name of an actual local healthcare facility should be used. A variety of databases exist on the Internet to identify the names of healthcare facilities in isolated geographic regions.[5]

The testing coordinator should develop a list of local healthcare facilities for callers to use in their background stories.

---

[5] For example: http://www.helplinedatabase.com/hospital-us/index.html lists all of the hospitals in the U.S. by state and county.

Chapter 4.
Training to Conduct a Test

Callers should be trained before they begin calling any public health agency participating in a test. This chapter outlines strategies that can be used by trainers to train callers and provides resources and materials for call training. A train-the-trainer approach is suggested for training large groups of callers. Training builds a caller's skill and confidence and minimizes errors that could potentially evoke a false alarm. Figure 4.1 highlights the three main aspects of training: preparing for a test, learning to debrief, and practice and observation.

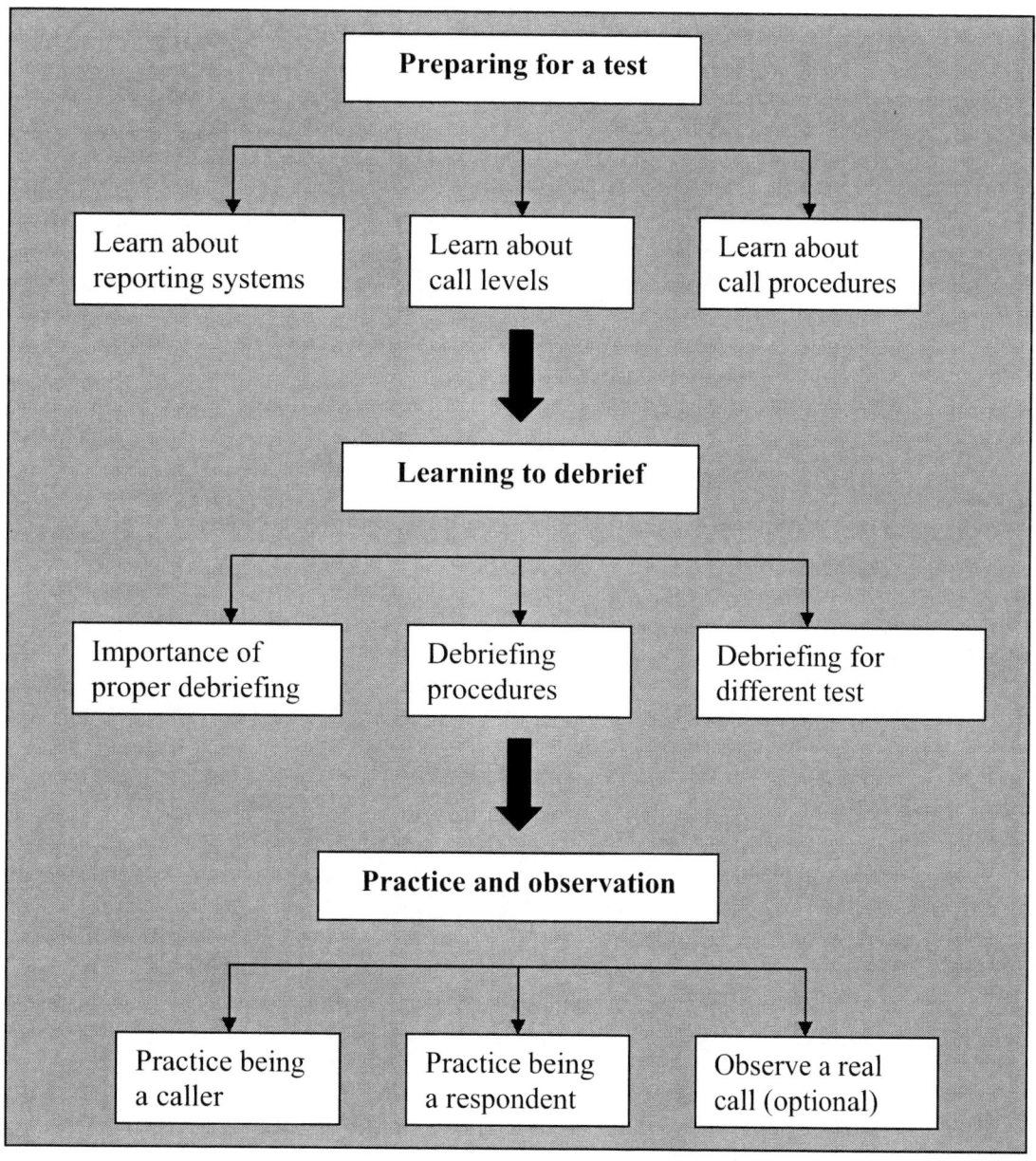

Figure 4.1 Framework for Test Training

TRAINER RESPONSIBILITIES

The trainer has several responsibilities, including
- Organizing and planning training sessions
- Preparing training materials
- Reviewing training materials with trainees
- Answering any questions trainees may have about testing procedures
- Conducting practice and observation calls with trainees.

Ideally, the trainer is someone who has participated as a caller in a test and thus has real-world experience with the procedures.

Organizing and planning training sessions involves setting a date(s) and time(s) for training session(s) and finding a location where the training session can take place. Usually a small conference room with a marker board or chalkboard is adequate. Trainers are responsible for making sure that trainees have training materials for the sessions.

Trainers should NOT provide trainees with an entire copy of this operations manual, which would most likely be overwhelming. Instead, chapters of the manual are recommended for training sessions (see below).

There are two two-hour training sessions:
- Session 1—Preparing for a test and learning to debrief
- Session 2—Practice and observation

These sessions can be conducted separately or together in a half-day seminar. The first session introduces trainees to public health disease reporting systems and terminology, and the general testing format of the tests provided in the manual. The second training session focuses on having trainees practice and observe calls. Trainees should be encouraged to play the role of both the caller and the respondent.

Trainers should begin each session by reviewing the objectives of the training session to trainees. Sessions should then follow the agendas included in Appendix B and C respectively. Sessions should end with a quick stocktaking in which trainees fill out a knowledge assessment and then discuss their answers with the trainer. Answers for the trainer to use to guide this discussion can be found in Appendix D. Trainers should be sure to leave time at the end of each training session for trainees to ask questions about testing procedures.

The next two sections describe these training sessions in more detail.

TRAINING SESSION 1: PREPARING FOR A TEST AND LEARNING TO DEBRIEF

The trainer should bring copies of the following items for trainees to the first training session:
- Appendix A (Terminology)
- Appendix B (Agenda, handouts, knowledge assessment)
- Appendix E (Testing template materials)
- Chapter 2 (Testing public health disease reporting systems)
- Chapter 5 (Testing phase)

The first training session is designed to introduce trainees to the tests and the testing procedures. It has four objectives:
- Introduce trainees to public health disease reporting systems and terminology
- Introduce trainees to the general testing format and testing levels
- Introduce trainees to debriefing and debriefing procedures
- Walk trainees through an example of each testing level.

After each objective, a chapter or Appendix of the training manual is highlighted. To accomplish each objective, the trainer should review these chapters of the manual with the trainees. During the session the trainer should be sure to highlight the terminology introduced in each chapter to trainees (Appendix A). Trainees should become familiar with the following concepts:
- Public health disease reporting system
- Testing level
- Action officer
- Warm transfer
- Lead-in
- Callback
- Debriefing

Appendix B contains a handout for callers, which provides them with the general steps necessary to conduct all calls. The trainer should walk trainees through examples of each level with respondents following the steps outlined in Chapter 5. It is important that trainees understand the basic steps involved in calls during the first training session; however, they will not actually practice calls until Session 2. The first training session should focus on having trainees understand the structure of calls for each test level. The trainer should end the session by reviewing the brief knowledge assessment (also provided in Appendix B) with trainees. The knowledge assessment is designed to ensure that trainees understand the basic concepts discussed in the training session and feel comfortable enough with the materials to begin practice calls. Answers to knowledge assessments can be found in Appendix D. The trainer should be sure to leave time for questions throughout the session. In particular, a generous amount of Q&A time should be allotted at the end of the session.

TRAINING SESSION 2: PRACTICE AND OBSERVATION

The trainer should bring copies of the following items for trainees to the second training session:

- Appendix C (Agenda, handouts, knowledge assessment)
- Appendix F (Data collection forms)
- Appendix G (CDC guidelines for public health disease reporting systems)

The practice training session is critical for trainees before they can begin placing real calls. The four primary goals of this session are to:

- Introduce "Quick Reference Sheets" to trainees (Appendix C)
- Introduce data collection forms to trainees (Appendix F)
- Provide trainees with experience placing calls
- Teach trainees strategies to overcoming roadblocks and problems during calls
- Answer any remaining questions trainees may have before making calls.

The purpose of Quick Reference Sheets is to provide trainees with informative and succinct "cheat sheets" to use while making their first few calls, until they are completely comfortable with making calls. The trainer should review these sheets with trainees at the beginning of the session and encourage trainees to use them while making calls. Sample data collection forms are also provided in Appendix F.

The trainer should begin by asking trainees to practice Level 1 calls. Initially the trainer should play the role of the responding public health agency. Trainees should be encouraged to role-play as if they were actually making a call. Trainees should also play the role of respondent to get a sense of how it feels to be a respondent to a call. The trainer should let trainees practice several calls each for which there are no problems to develop a general feeling the calling process.

Level 4 tests require the most amount of practice—probably more than a single practice session. Trainees may wish to conduct several real Level 3 calls and then have another practice session dedicated to Level 4 calls before placing an actual Level 4 call.

After trainees have practiced making calls on all levels, the trainer should play the role of the respondent and begin to introduce roadblocks during practice calls. Several common problems and roadblocks are suggested below; trainers should also feel free to draw upon their own experience in developing practice roadblocks. The trainer should introduce roadblocks during each of the major components of a call (e.g., call initiation, reaching an action officer debriefing).

Examples of practice roadblocks include:

Call initiation
- The hesitant receptionist—a receptionist who refuses to transfer the caller or let the caller leave a message without more information.

- The confusing call system—a call system in which callers are transferred from call station to call station, with each requesting information about the call

Reaching an action officer
- The concerned action officer—an action officer who is worried that the call is being placed by a terrorist trying to find weaknesses in the public health agency's response system
- The angry action officer—an action officer who is angry that the call he or she received is just a test
- The missing action officer—an action officer who never returns a call
- The questioning action officer—an action officer who would like to know how he/she performed on the test

Debriefing
- The disconnected call—a caller gets disconnected before he or she can properly debrief the action officer
- The confused action officer—an action officer who doesn't seem to understand the test.

Chapter 5.
Conducting a Test

After a test has been chosen and planned and training is complete, testing is ready to begin. This chapter outlines a set of tools and templates that callers can use in conducting tests. Figure 5.1 presents a framework for conducting a test.

All calls in all levels begin with similar initiating procedures. The only difference is whether or not a disguise is used in the lead-in. After reaching an action officer:

- Level 1 callback respondents are immediately debriefed. Nothing else is requested of them.
- Level 2 callback respondents are immediately debriefed; however, they are asked a series of procedural questions.
- Level 3 callback respondents are immediately debriefed and then asked a series of procedural and content questions.
- Level 4 callbacks are not immediately debriefed but instead are first given a concerning case report. Respondents are debriefed immediately after they describe to the callers the initial procedures they should take.

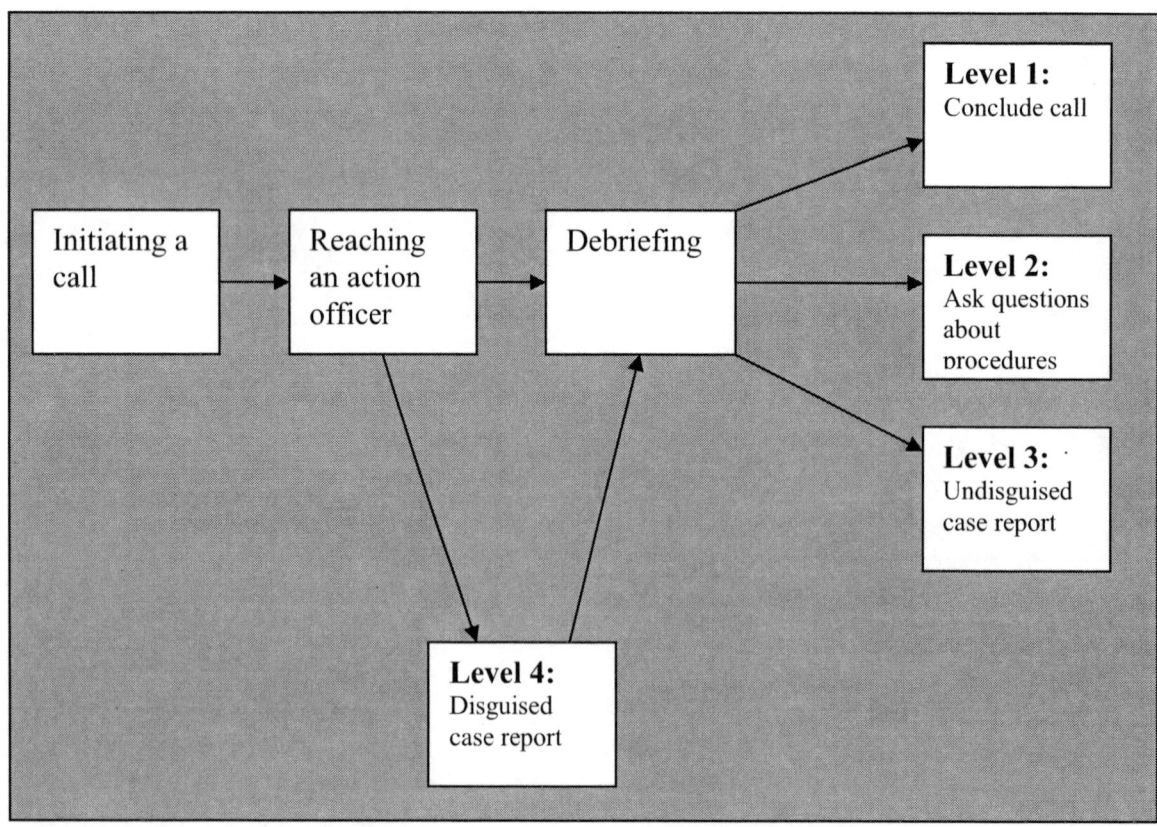

Figure 5.1 Framework for Conducting a Test

INITIATING A CALL

This section outlines the steps for initiating a call for all of the call levels. Template scripts for call initiation can be found in Appendix E.

Step 1
Record date and time immediately prior to placing the call.

Step 2
Call the public health agency using an appropriate number (main public health agency telephone number, communicable/infectious disease department number, after-hours hotline, etc).

Step 3
Upon contact with the public health agency, use an appropriate lead-in message. The call may be answered by:

1. Public health agency switchboard operator or answering service (main public health agency operator, division/department/bureau operator, emergency/after hours operator, etc.)
   o Use a "call initiation lead-in" script (examples are in Appendix E) as a template for what to say to the operator. Appendix E contains samples of scripts that involve using a disguise and scripts that do not involve a disguise. If the call involves using a disguise, it is important that lead-in script be changed for every call.

2. Public health agency answering machine/voicemail (main public health agency message recording system, division/department/bureau message system, individual action officer message recording system, etc.)
   o Leave a message for the action officer requesting a callback.

3. Public health agency action officer (epidemiologist, bioterrorism coordinator, public health nurse, etc).
   o Follow the scripts for reaching an action officer for the appropriate test level.

4. No answer (dead-end phone system with no ability to leave a message and no options, such as instructions for reaching an alternative number or paging system)
   o Record the call as a failure.

REACHING AN ACTION OFFICER

After reaching an action officer, follow the following steps:

Step 1
Record the date and time of the contact.

<u>Step 2</u>

Ask the respondent if he or she is the appropriate person to handle a case report involving an infectious disease.

> *If the answer is "<u>No</u>,"* ask to be transferred to the appropriate person or have the appropriate person make a callback and repeat Steps 1 and 2.
>
> *If the answer is "<u>Yes</u>,"* proceed with debriefing for the appropriate test level.

<u>Step 3</u>

For all calls except Level 4, begin debriefing. For Level 4 calls, present the action officer with a case report (templates are in Appendix E) and ask the appropriate questions. Go into Level 4 debriefing immediately after the action officer answers the questions.

DEBRIEFING

Level 1

> <u>Step 1</u>
>
> Upon verifying you have reached an appropriate action officer, immediately debrief the respondent, using the Level 1 Debriefing script in Appendix E as a template.
>
> <u>Step 2</u>
>
> Record the following information:
> a) Title/position of the action officer
> c) Title/position of individual notifying the action officer
> d) Date/time when the action officer was first notified (if you have left a message)
> e) Additional comments and notes detailing the call.
>
> <u>Step 3</u>
> End call.

Level 2

> <u>Step 1</u>
>
> Upon verifying you have reached an appropriate action officer, immediately debrief the respondent, using the Level 2 debriefing script in Appendix E as a template.
>
> <u>Step 2</u>
>
> As in a Level 1 call, record the following information:
> a) Title/position of the action officer
> b) Title/position of individual notifying the action officer
> c) Date/time when the action officer was first notified (if you have left a message)
> d) Additional comments and notes detailing the call.
>
> <u>Step 3</u>
>
> Ask the following callback questions and record the responses:
> a) How does your public health agency normally triage case reports?

b) What next steps would you take?
c) What additional information on cases would you ask for?
d) Who would you routinely notify?

Step 4 (*optional*)
If the respondent who contacted the caller does not appear to be an appropriate action officer, the caller may ask the respondent to contact a more appropriate action officer and have that person call back.

Step 5
End call.

Level 3

Step 1
Upon verifying you have reached an appropriate action officer, immediately debrief the respondent, using the Level 3 debriefing script in Appendix E as a template.

Step 2
As in a Level 1 call, record the following information:
a) Title/position of the action officer
b) Title/position of individual notifying action officer
c) Date/time when action officer was first notified (if you have left a message)
d) Additional comments and notes detailing the call

Step 3
Ask the caller to respond to a case report, such as that contained in Appendix E.
a) Choose one case (for example, botulism, anthrax, or smallpox)
b) Read the case report to the action officer
c) Important: ensure that the action officer understands that this phone call is only a test and not a real case.

Record the answers to the following questions:
a) How does your public health agency normally triage case reports?
b) What next steps would you take?
c) What additional information on cases would you ask for?
d) Who would you routinely notify?

Step 4 (*optional*)
If the respondent who contacted the caller does not appear to be an appropriate action officer, the caller may ask the respondent to contact a more appropriate action officer and have that person call back.
a) Important: the action officer must inform his contact that the phone call and the case report are not real.
b) Repeat Step 3 for the next contacted individual.

Step 5
End call.

Level 4
Step 1
Upon verifying you have reached an appropriate action officer, do not inform the action officer of the test. Rather, proceed with a case report (templates for case reports are in Appendix E).
a) Choose one case (for example, botulism, anthrax, or smallpox)
b) Read the case report to the action officer, maintaining the guise of a real caller.
Begin debriefing immediately if:
a) The action officer can no longer handle the case (due, for example, to stress and/or inexperience).
b) The action officer wishes to break telephone contact (for example, place you on hold or call you back).

Under no circumstances should you break telephone contact with the action officer without having revealed the call to be a test and not a real case. If at any time you begin to lose control of the conversation (for example, due to reasons such as a) or b) above), immediately inform the action officer that the case report is not real and proceed to Step 3.

Step 2
Allow the action officer to respond to the case. Answer all questions posed to you as best you can (again, using the case report clinical questions and answers as a guide—see Appendix E). Additionally, use the following questions as a guide or as prompts to test the action officer's capacity:
a) Is there any more information you need from me?
b) What should I do next?
c) What are the next steps you are going to take?
d) Is there anyone else at the public health agency who should be hearing this?

Step 3
Upon gathering the information in Step 2, inform the action officer that the call is not real. Use the Level 4 debriefing script as a guide (Appendix E).

Step 4
As in a Level 1 call, record the following information:
a) Title/position of the action officer
b) Title/position of individual notifying action officer
c) Date/time when action officer was first notified (if you have left a message)
d) Additional comments and notes detailing the call.

Step 5 (*optional*)

If the respondent who contacted the caller does not appear to be an appropriate action officer, the caller may ask the respondent to contact a more appropriate action officer and have that person call back.

a) Important: the action officer must inform the contact that the phone call and the case report are not real. Ensure that this has occurred.

b) Allow the action officer to "educate" the new contact regarding the revealed false case report.

c) Repeat steps 2, 3, and 4.

<u>Step 6</u>
End call.

Chapter 6.
Assessing Test Performance

Once a test has been completed, procedures should be in place for evaluating the performance of the participating public health agency and providing constructive feedback in the form of an after-action report. An *after-action report* summarizes the public health agency's performance in the test. A sample after-action report is provided in Appendix I.

The testing coordinator is responsible for generating these reports. The testing coordinator should compile the results of both the quantitative and qualitative aspects of the test. Quantitative aspects of the test include the median response time that respondents took to return the calls, the percentage of calls in which an appropriate action officer performed the first callback, and the percentage or number of failed calls. Qualitative aspects include an assessment of the respondent's knowledge of the public health agency's protocols that relate to its disease reporting system and the quality of respondents' responses to case reports. Reports should end with an assessment of the overall quality of the public health agency's response using performance criterion established by the CDC (see Appendix G). The framework for these activities is provided in Figure 6.1.

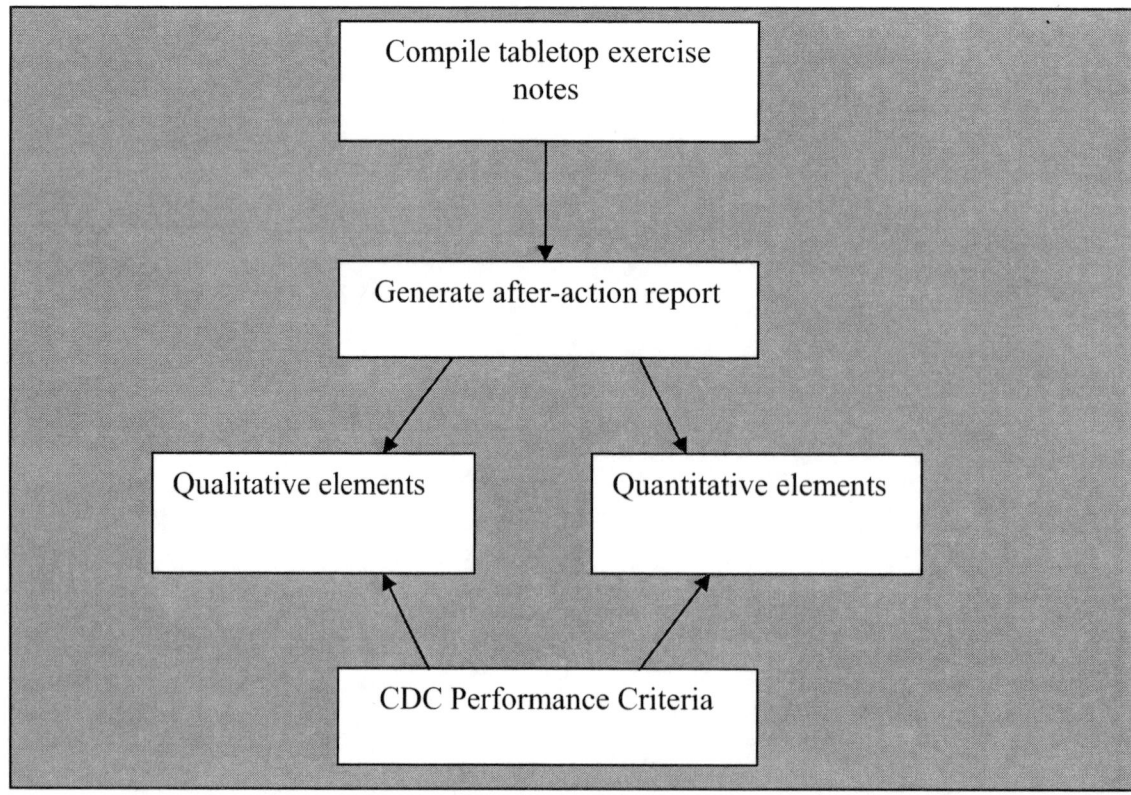

Figure 6.1 Framework for Assessing Test Performance

PERFORMANCE CRITERIA

This section outlines performance criteria that public health agencies can use to evaluate their performance for each testing level. These criteria provide a set of consistent and standardized measures that can be used to regularly evaluate public health disease reporting systems. They were created based on standards developed by the CDC (see Appendix G). Every testing level has specific performance criteria. Appendix F contains sample data collection forms that can be used by callers to obtain information during calls for each of these measures.

Availability of telephone number

Four performance criteria should be collected prior to making any calls to a public health agency. These criteria relate to the availability of an appropriate telephone number for disease reporting. They include (Table 6.1):

- Single number available for all calls day or night (yes/no)
- Telephone number available through local directory assistance (yes/no)
- Single telephone number well publicized (e.g., same number found in more than one source) (yes/no)
- Total number of telephone numbers at public health agency related to public health disease reporting.

The CDC recommends that all public health agencies have a single well-publicized number available on directory assistance for public health disease reporting systems. Having many telephone numbers that could potentially be used for public health disease reporting creates confusion. If the same telephone number for public health disease reporting can be found for a public health agency in more than one source (e.g., on the Internet and in the local directory assistance), it is considered well publicized.

Call initiation

There are eight performance criteria that relate to call initiation (Table 6.1):

- Percentage of calls answered within 5 rings
- Length of wait time on hold in minutes
- Percentage of calls transferred in 5 rings
- Percentage of calls that were *warm transfers*
- Percentage of calls that were *dead end* calls
- Percent of calls responded to by an appropriate action officer on first callback or transfer
- Length of wait for call back in minutes
- Percentage of calls that received a callback in 30 minutes or less

All of these measures listed above can be assessed in testing Levels 1–4. The preferred mode of transfer is a "warm transfer" whereby callers are directly transferred to action officers. Calls should never reach dead ends.

Table 6.1 Summary of Quantitative Performance Criteria for Tests

Performance Criterion	Type of variable	Test Level		
		1	2	3–4
Single number available for all calls day or night	yes/no	●	●	●
Telephone number available through local directory assistance	yes/no	●	●	●
Single telephone number well publicized (e.g., same number found in more than one source)	yes/no	●	●	●
Total number of telephone numbers at public health agency related to public health disease reporting	Continuous	●	●	●
Percentage of calls answered within 5 rings	Percentage	●	●	●
Length of wait time on hold in minutes	Continuous	●	●	●
Percentage of calls transferred in 5 rings	Percentage	●	●	●
Percentage of calls that were *warm transfers*	Percentage	●	●	●
Percentage of calls that were *dead end* calls	Percentage	●	●	●
Percent of calls responded to by an appropriate action officer on first callback or transfer	Percentage	●	●	●
Length of wait for call back in minutes	Continuous	●	●	●
Percentage of calls that received a callback in 30 minutes or less	Percentage	●	●	●
Percentage of calls where action officer knew if their public health agency has a formal triage protocol for concerning case reports	Percentage		●	●
Percentage of calls where action officer was aware of whether public health agency has the ability to record calls for quality assurance	Percentage		●	●
Percentage of calls where action officer knew about surge capacity for the public health agency's public health disease reporting system	Percentage		●	●
Percentage of calls where action officer knew whether or not he or she could initiate a three-way call for concerning case reports	Percentage		●	●
Percentage of calls where action officer knew whether or not a backup action officer was available during the time of the call	Percentage		●	●
Percentage of calls where action officer determined the disease being discussed in the case report without being told by the caller	Percentage			●
Percentage of calls where action officer discussed personal protective equipment with the caller without first being probed	Percentage			●
Percentage of calls where action officer asked for more case details after hearing case report	Percentage			●

Procedural knowledge

There are five performance measures that evaluate a respondent's procedural knowledge (Table 6.2):

- Percentage of calls where action officer knew if their public health agency has a formal triage protocol for concerning case reports
- Percentage of calls where action officer was aware of whether the public health agency has the ability to record calls for quality assurance
- Percentage of calls where action officer knew about the public health agency's surge capacity for the disease reporting system
- Percentage of calls where action officer knew whether or not he or she could initiate a three-way call for concerning case reports
- Percentage of calls where action officer knew whether or not a backup action officer was available during the time of the call

These measures can be assessed only in testing Levels 2–4.

Content knowledge

There are three performance criteria that evaluate a respondent's content knowledge (Table 6.2):

- Percentage of calls where action officer determined the disease being discussed in the case report without being told by the caller
- Percentage of calls where action officer discussed personal protective equipment with the caller without first being probed
- Percentage of calls where action officer asked for more case details after hearing case report.

These measures can be assessed only during testing Levels 3–4.

Quantitative measures like the ones discussed in "Procedural knowledge" and "Content knowledge" above are useful, but do not provide a sufficient level of detail for testing Levels 2–4. These levels involve conversations that can provide useful qualitative information. Table 6.2 identifies qualitative measures that can be used to evaluate public health agencies. These measures should be used as examples of the type of qualitative data that callers should try to extract from respondents. Callers should take notes during the calls to collect this data.

Callers for Levels 2–4 should probe respondents' knowledge of their public health agency's phone triage protocol for concerning case reports. It is important for the caller to determine whether or not the action officer understands how case reports are triaged in that public health agency. Callers should also ascertain whether or not respondents know about their public health agency's disease reporting system's capability, both in terms of surge capacity and three-way calls. Finally, respondents to Levels 2–4 call should understand their department's procedures for backups.

Table 6.2 Summary of Qualitative Performance Criteria for Tests

Description	Performance criterion
Action officer's knowledge of the public health agency's phone triage protocol for concerning disease reports	1. Was the action officer able to describe the public health agency's protocol? 2. Was the description clear or confusing? 3. How detailed was the description? 4. Did the action officer know whom he or she would contact next?
Action officer's knowledge of the public health agency's public health disease reporting system's capabilities	1. What did the action officer know about his or her disease reporting system's surge capacity? 2. What did the action officer know about establishing a three-way call? 3. Could he/she establish a three-way call if necessary?
Action officer's knowledge of backup availability	1. Who is the backup on duty if the action officer is not available? 2. Does the action officer know the name and contact information for the backup? 3. How long would it take the backup to respond to a call?
Action officer's content knowledge	1. Did the action officer struggle to identify the disease described in the case report? 2. What questions did he/she ask? 3. Were they good questions? 4. Was the action officer's feedback helpful?
Action officer's response to case report	1. Did the action officer ask for the caller's name and contact information? 2. Did the action officer have a clear response plan for moving forward? 3. How long was the call? 4. Did the caller feel satisfied at the end of the call that the action officer was in control of the situation?

Callers testing Levels 3–4 should probe respondents' clinical knowledge to determine whether they would be able to respond to the report presented to them. Callers should record whether they feel that the respondent has a strong grasp of what needs to be done and what steps need to be taken to ensure that the situation remains under control.

GENERATING AN AFTER-ACTION REPORT

Compilation of test results should relate directly to the ultimate goal of the tests, which is to ensure that public health agencies have a sufficient level of proficiency to respond to public health disease reports as outlined by the CDC. Results should be presented in a way that is succinct and easy to understand and provides a set of reasonable benchmarks.

The easiest way to provide public health agencies with this type of feedback is to generate an after-action report that summarizes their performance on the test. The summary measures outlined in Tables 6.1 and 6.2 can be used to generate an after-action report. An after-action report should have four components:
- Summary of exercise (how many calls were made, times of day in which calls were made, when calls began and ended, etc.)
- Summary of quantitative measures (outline performance on measures discussed in Table 6.1)
- Summary of qualitative measures (brief discussion of respondent responses to tests—Table 6.2)
- Areas for improvement.

A sample after-action report can be found in Appendix I.

Chapter 7.
Establishing a Regular System of Testing

Public health disease reporting systems are critical parts of the infrastructure of all public health agencies. To ensure that these systems are functioning properly, it is necessary to evaluate them regularly. The CDC recommends that public health agencies develop regular, formal, standardized protocols of unannounced testing for their public health disease reporting systems and that these systems be tested at least annually.

The test templates discussed in this manual are meant to assist public health agencies in achieving this aim. Public health agencies need to regularly test their public health disease reporting systems for a variety of reasons, including
- Staff turnover
- New or revised procedures or protocols
- New telephone systems or numbers
- Changes in answering services or operators.

Figure 7.1 outlines a framework for establishing a regular testing protocol. Establishing such a system begins with establishing a baseline level of testing proficiency that can be used as a comparison for later tests. Tests can be used to regularly evaluate and improve the system allowing for continuous quality improvement.

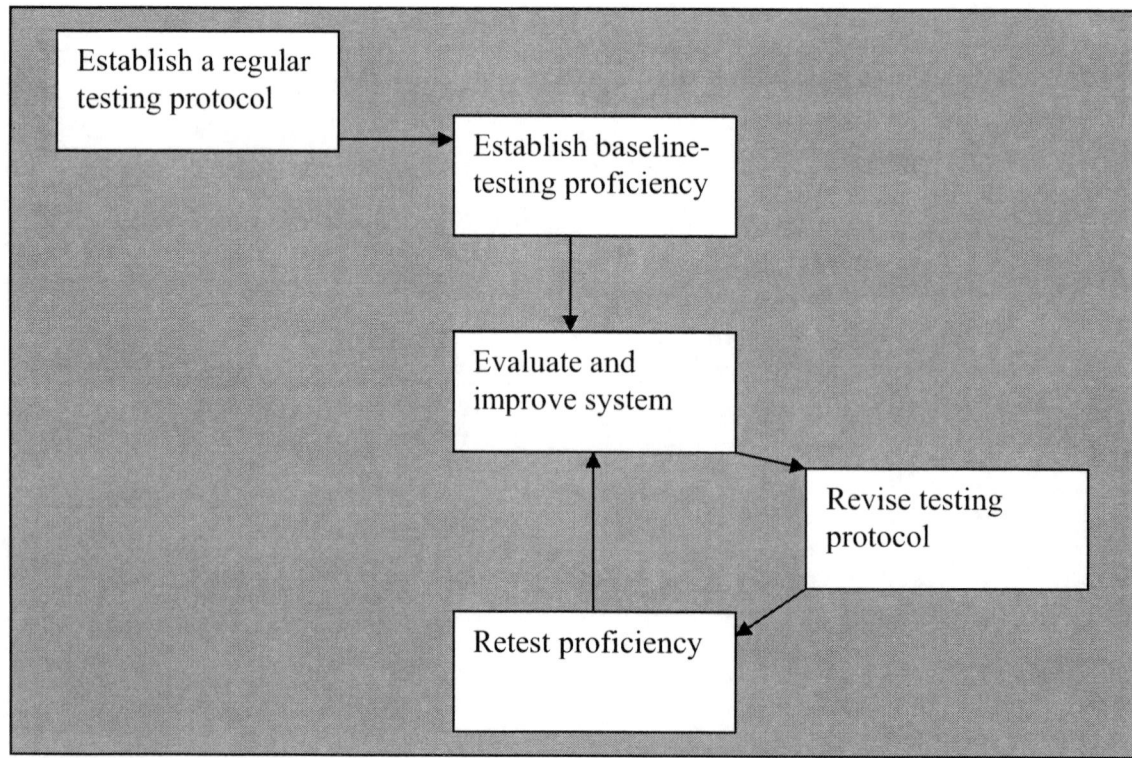

Figure 7.1 Framework for Establishing a Regular System of Testing

CONTINUOUS QUALITY IMPROVEMENT

Not all public health agencies are ready for completely unannounced tests of their public health disease reporting systems. Recognizing that fact, this manual outlines a number of different testing levels that meet public health agencies where they are with their current public health disease reporting systems. Public health agency leadership is encouraged to use these tests to continuously improve and retest their systems.

Continuous quality improvement (CQI) is a term used to describe a comprehensive management philosophy that emphasizes the continuous improvement of work processes for improved outcomes. Public health agencies can use the tests outlined in this manual as part of an overall CQI strategy to improve their public health disease reporting systems.

Public health agencies are encouraged to begin by ensuring that their public health disease reporting system
- Can receive calls 24/7
- Has one telephone number for calls day or night
- Has a well-publicized telephone number known by all healthcare workers.

Once these basic steps have been met, public health agencies are encouraged to test their public health disease reporting system as part of a regular performance measurement and improvement system. The testing agency and the public health agency or departments that it is testing should establish a routine system of testing with the goal of continually improving the system and ensuring that changes in staffing or public health agency infrastructure are not detrimental to the system.

State public health agencies that have authority over LPHAs may wish to establish a rule that LPHAs can expect their public health disease reporting systems to be tested each year during an unannounced time period. These tests can be self-tests; however, they are likely to be more valid if they are conducted by an agency other than the public health agency being tested.

Public health agencies with 24/7 public health disease reporting systems that have never been tested or that are new in development should begin by testing their public health agency with an announced Level 1 test that does not involve the use of any disguises. Once the system appears to function well enough to handle these tests, the public health agency should consider moving to either a Level 2 test or a Level 1 test that is unannounced or that involves the use of disguises or both.

It is up to the discretion of public health agency leadership to decide which of the 21 tests described in Table 3.1 to use to test their public health agency. These tests progress in terms of realism and difficulty. Public health agencies that feel that they have very advanced public health disease reporting systems should consider beginning with an unannounced Level 3 test that involves the use of disguises. If the public health agency is able to complete this test it should move to a Level 4 test in the next round of testing.

The idea is to continually move up the scale of realism and difficulty in the tests until your public health agency is able to respond in a timely and appropriate manner to the most difficult and realistic of the tests (e.g., completely unannounced Level 4 tests). Once this goal is achieved you should regularly (e.g., at least annually) test your public health agency with this test to ensure that the system continues to function properly. This process ensures a CQI strategy for continually improving your public health agency's public health disease reporting system.

When choosing a test, it is best to first choose one you feel is below the level of your public health agency. This will avoid the risk of giving a test at your public health agency that may frustrate the staff or—worse—accidentally initiate a real public health response that could have negative consequences.

MOVING FORWARD

As technology changes, so will public health disease reporting systems. Many public health agencies have established or are in the process of establishing computerized or Internet based public health disease reporting systems for health care workers to use for case reporting. As these changes take hold in public health agencies, new strategies will need to be developed to continually evaluate them.

Nothing, however, can replace the value of a telephone call in which real-time information can be relayed from health care professionals on the front lines to public health agency staff. Therefore it is likely that future public health disease reporting systems will continue to utilize telephones for the most urgent of cases.

Appendix A.
Terminology

Action officer – *Public health professional* whose responsibility is to respond to concerning case reports placed by health care workers to public health disease reporting systems. Action officers can be public health agency directors, *epidemiologists*, *bioterrorism coordinators*, doctors, nurses, etc. Action officers should have sufficient training, and clinical knowledge to be able to respond appropriately to 80% of all the calls made to a public health agency.

After-action report – A report summarizing the results of a public health agency's public health disease reporting test.

Background story – Information used during *call initiation* that presents a plausible scenario for calls that involve using a disguise.

Baseline – A unit or measurement taken at a specific time point that can be used as a comparison for later measurements of the same phenomenon.

Bioterrorism – The intentional release of a biological agent into an environment with the intent to harm the living beings in that environment. Abbreviated as BT.

Bioterrorism coordinator – A public health agency employee in charge of managing their department's planning and response to a *bioterrorism* emergency.

Callback – A call received from an action officer as a follow-up to a message from a caller.

Caller – Individuals working for the testing agency responsible for placing test calls and recording the responses.

Call initiation – The act of placing a call to a public health agency to report a *concerning case*.

Call schedule – A calendar that identifies the dates and times for calls as well as the caller(s) responsible for placing the calls.

Case report – A report placed to a public health agency via telephone, fax, or e-mail from a healthcare professional regarding a case with a *reportable disease*, a *disease cluster*, or a *concerning case* that may require the attention of public health professionals.

Concerning case – A case that could potentially represent a severe public health threat.

Continuous quality improvement – A term used to describe a comprehensive management philosophy, emphasizing the continuous improvement of work processes for improved outcomes.

Dead end – The end of an automated call system in which the caller is not given the opportunity to leave a message or provided with another telephone number to call in an emergency.

Debriefing – The act of revealing the nature of the test, its goals, and its sponsors, including the names of the exercise coordinator and the people at the public health agency who provided their consent. Debriefing is the point at which the caller tells the action officer responding to a call that the call is only a test and requires no further action.

Detection – Occurs when the staff members at a public health agency being tested become aware of the test.

Disease cluster – A cluster of patients in a defined geographic area experiencing similar signs and symptoms of an unexpected or concerning nature.

Disguise – The use of role-playing during a call to enhance the realism of the call. A disguise typically involves a caller pretending to be a healthcare worker calling a public health agency about a concerning case.

Epidemiologist – An investigator who studies the occurrence of disease or other health-related conditions or events in defined populations. Disease control is often also considered to be a task for the epidemiologist, especially in certain specialized fields, such as malaria epidemiology.

Evaluation phase – Phase after testing that involves evaluating the tested public health agency in terms of speed and quality of response.

Lead-in – A message that moves a call from a reception desk or answering service to an action officer. It is composed of the caller's name and hospital affiliation, and the request to speak with someone about a patient—a *concerning case*. The lead-in never includes any case details.

Local public health agency – A term used to signify all public health agencies below the state level (e.g., county, municipal, etc.).

Menu approach – An approach to developing *call schedules* that allows callers to choose call times from a menu of options, thereby ensuring that all applicable time periods are covered in the test.

Planning phase – Phase of exercise development in which the supervisor chooses a public health agency to test, chooses an appropriate test, identifies or hires staff, purchases materials required to conduct tests, plans testing activities, etc.

Public health disease reporting system – A system developed by a public health agency to receive case reports from health care workers, usually by telephone.

Public health professional – A person who works for a public health agency who has knowledge and training in public health.

Proficiency test – A tool to monitor the performance and readiness of individuals, agencies, or organizations. The goal is to ensure that tasks are being performed at an acceptable level. Proficiency tests are also called operation readiness inspections, clinical audits, response exercises, performance drills, vigilance tests, and preparedness tests.

Reportable disease – A disease with public health importance that healthcare professionals are required to report to their LPHA.

Test coordinator – The individual in charge of planning and coordinating tests, ensuring staff is properly trained, and answering any questions that callers or respondents might have about the exercises.

Testing Levels – Four separate proficiency tests of increasing levels of difficulty, developed to test the proficiency of public health disease reporting systems.

Testing agency – The agency or organization responsible for conducting a test of a public health agency's public health disease reporting system.

Testing phase – Phase during which a public health agency's public health disease reporting systems are tested by the testing agency.

Testing supervisor – The individual with the authority to conduct a test who provides supervision for the entire testing period.

Trainer – The individual responsible for planning, coordinating, and running training sessions for new callers.

Training phase – Phase of exercise development where staff at the testing agency are trained to conduct proficiency tests of public health disease reporting systems.

Warm transfer – A call that is transferred directly from a receptionist or answering service at a public health agency to an appropriate action officer.

Appendix B.
Training Session 1 Materials

Training Session 1: Preparing for a Test and Learning to Debrief

Agenda

I.   Introduction to public health disease reporting systems (refer to Chapter 2 handout)
   a. Purpose
   b. Structure

II.   General testing format
   a. Initiating a call
      i. Lead-in
      ii. Callbacks
   b. Reaching an action officer
   c. Debriefing

III.   Advanced notification
   a. Preplanned tests
   b. Unscheduled tests
   c. Unannounced test

IV.   Use of disguises
   a. Why use disguises
   b. How to avoid problems using disguises

V.   Description of testing levels
   a. Level 1
   b. Level 2
   c. Level 3
   d. Level 4

VI.   Step-by-step examples of calls (refer to Chapter 5 handout)
   a. Walk through a sample call from each test level from start to finish
   b. Review terminology (Appendix A)
   c. Question/answer session

Training Session 1: Preparing for a Test and Learning to Debrief

Knowledge Assessment

1. What is the purpose of public health disease reporting systems?

2. How often should public health agencies test their public health disease reporting systems?

3. What is an "action officer" and what roles and responsibilities does he/she have?

4. What are the three major elements of all tests?

5. Why is responding to case reports as soon as possible so important?

6. What form of communication is the primary means for public health disease reporting systems and why?

7. What is the maximum amount of time that the CDC recommends for action officers to respond to concerning case reports?

8. What is a lead-in?

9. What are the major elements of a proper debriefing?

10. Describe ways in which calls that involve the use of a disguise differ from calls that do not involve a disguise.

Appendix C.
Training Session 2 Materials

Training Session 2: Practice and Observation

Agenda

I.   Introduction to Quick Reference Sheets
        a. Initiating a call
        b. Reaching an action officer
        c. Debriefing

II.   Practice calls with role playing
        a. Trainees practicing being callers
        b. Trainees practicing being respondents

III.   Practice calls with roadblocks
        a. Call initiation problems
        b. Problems after reaching an action officer
        c. Problems during debriefing

IV.   Question/answer session

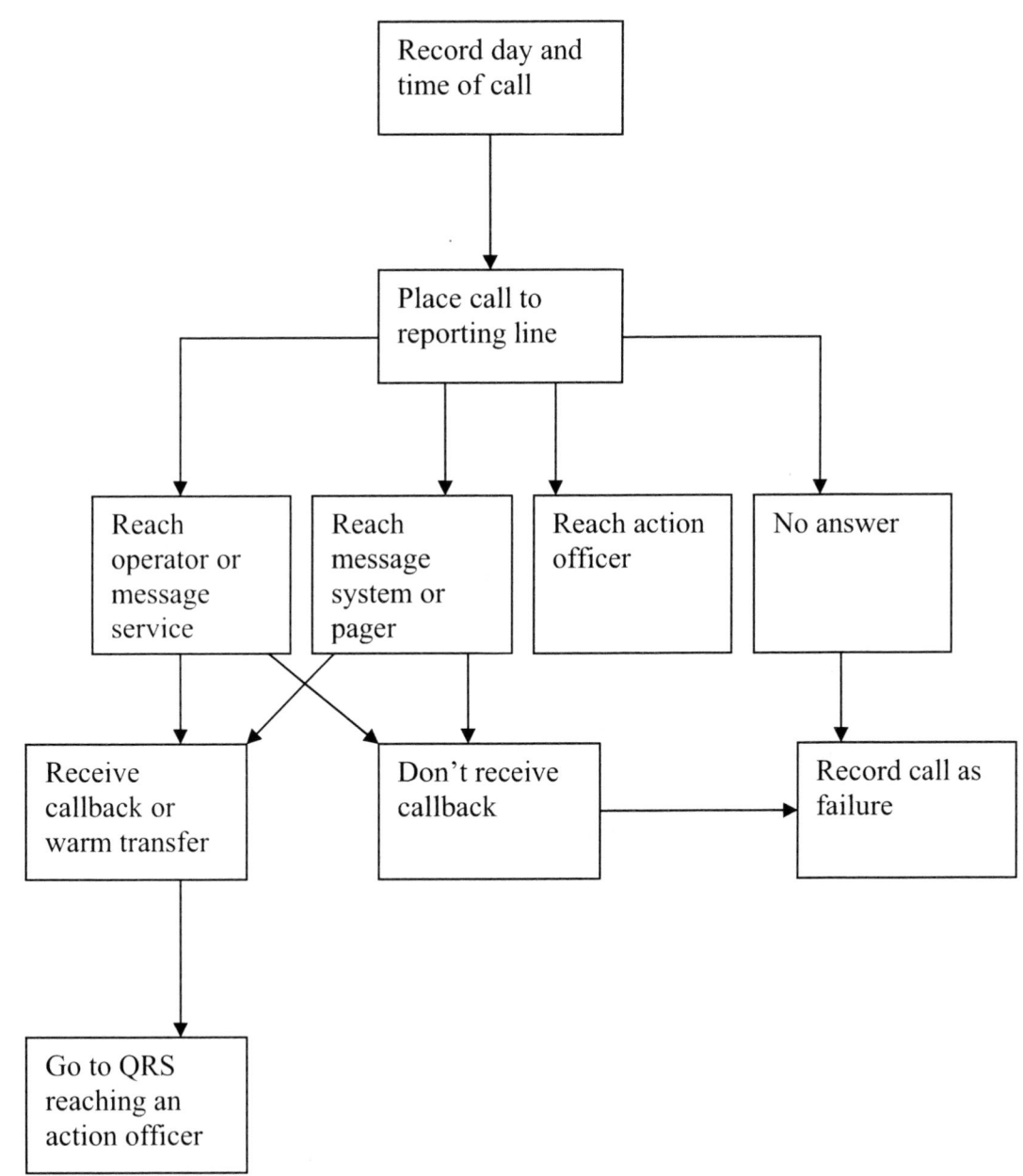

Quick Reference Sheet:
Initiating a Call

Record day and time of call

Place call to reporting line

Reach operator or message service

Reach message system or pager

Reach action officer

No answer

Receive callback or warm transfer

Don't receive callback

Record call as failure

Go to QRS reaching an action officer

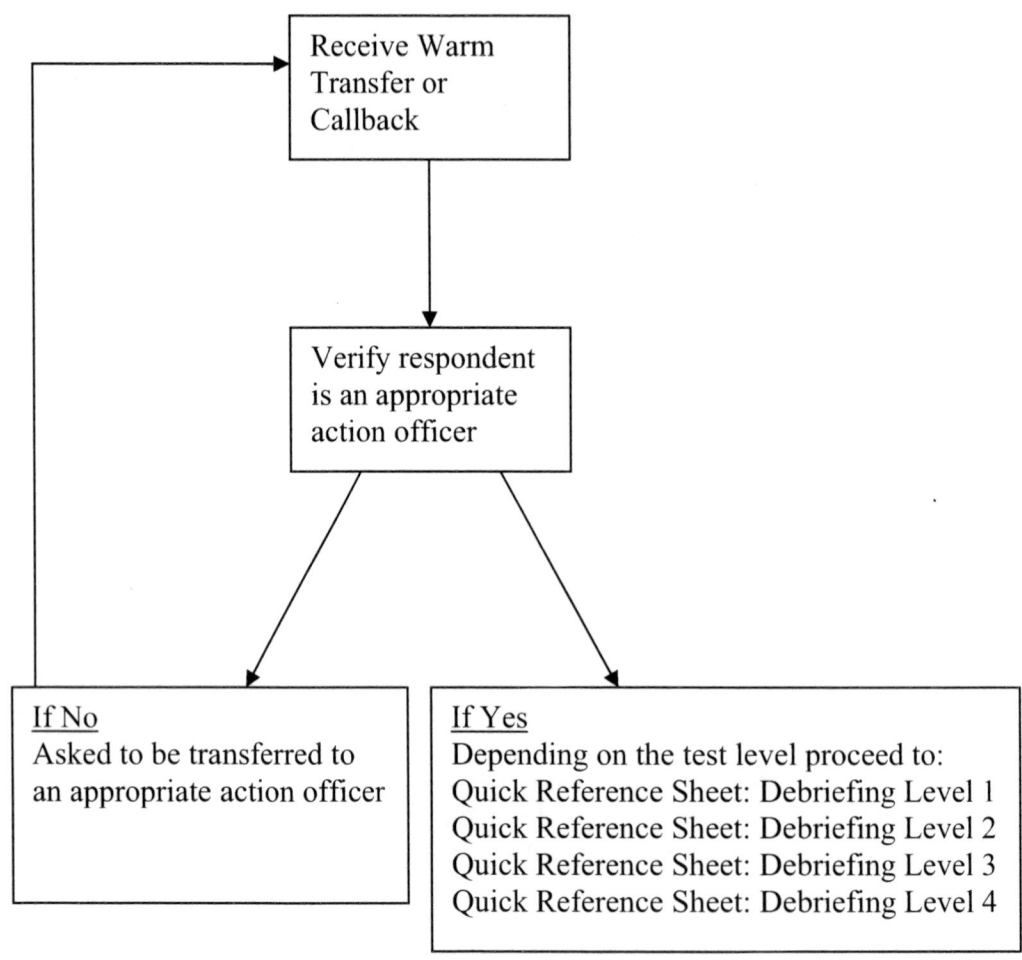

Receive Warm Transfer or Callback

Verify respondent is an appropriate action officer

If No
Asked to be transferred to an appropriate action officer

If Yes
Depending on the test level proceed to:
Quick Reference Sheet: Debriefing Level 1
Quick Reference Sheet: Debriefing Level 2
Quick Reference Sheet: Debriefing Level 3
Quick Reference Sheet: Debriefing Level 4

Quick Reference Sheet:
Debriefing Level 1

1. Verify you have reached an action officer
a) Ask the respondent if they are responsible for receiving urgent case reports

2. Debrief action officer
a) Inform action officer that call is not real
b) Ensure that the action officer understands no further response is necessary
c) Tell the caller who consented for the test and who they can contact

3. Record the following data:
a) Time and date verified action officer was reached
b) Title/position of action officer
c) Title/position of individual notifying action officer (if applicable)
d) Time and date action officer was first notified
e) Additional comments

4. Conclude Call
a) Ask if the action officer has any remaining questions
b) Thank the action officer for their time

Quick Reference Sheet:
Debriefing Level 2

1. Verify you have reached an action officer
a) Ask the respondent if they are responsible for receiving urgent case reports

2. Debrief action officer
a) Inform action officer that call is not real
b) Ensure that the action officer understands no further response is necessary
c) Tell the caller who consented for the test and who they can contact

3. Record the following data:
a) Time and date verified action officer was reached
b) Title/position of action officer
c) Title/position of individual notifying action officer (if applicable)
d) Time and date action officer was first notified
e) Additional comments

4. Ask questions about procedural knowledge
a) Does your HD have a formal procedure for triaging concerning case reports
b) Is your HD able to record calls for quality assurance purposes
c) Is your HD able to hand a large surge in reporting of concerning cases
d) Could you initiate a 3-way call right now if necessary?
e) Is there a backup action officer on call that could respond to this call?

5. Conclude Call
a) Ask if the action officer has any remaining questions
b) Thank the action officer for their time

Quick Reference Sheet: Debriefing Level 3

1. Verify you have reached an action officer
a) Ask the respondent if they are responsible for receiving urgent case reports

2. Debrief action officer
a) Inform action officer that call is not real
b) Ensure that the action officer understands no further response is necessary
c) Tell the caller who consented for the test and who they can contact

3. Record the following data:
a) Time and date verified action officer was reached
b) Title/position of action officer
c) Title/position of individual notifying action officer (if applicable)
d) Time and date action officer was first notified
e) Additional comments

4. Ask questions about procedural knowledge
a) Does your HD have a formal procedure for triaging concerning case reports
b) Is your HD able to record calls for quality assurance purposes
c) Is your HD able to hand a large surge in reporting of concerning cases
d) Could you initiate a 3-way call right now if necessary?
e) Is there a backup action officer on call that could respond to this call?

5. Present simulated case report and record:
a) Was the action officer able to identify the disease in the case report?
b) Did the action officer offer advice the caller advice (e.g., use of PPE, etc.)
c) Did the action officer ask for more information about the case

5. Conclude Call
a) Ask if the action officer has any remaining questions
b) Thank the action officer for their time

Quick Reference Sheet:
Debriefing Level 4

1. Verify you have reached an action officer
a) Ask the respondent if they are responsible for receiving urgent case reports

2. Present simulated case report and record (before debriefing):
a) Was the action officer able to identify the disease in the case report?
b) Did the action officer offer advice the caller advice (e.g., use of PPE, etc.)
c) Did the action officer ask for more information about the case

3. Debrief action officer
a) Inform action officer that call is not real
b) Ensure that the action officer understands no further response is necessary
c) Tell the caller who consented for the test and who they can contact

4. Record the following data:
a) Time and date verified action officer was reached
b) Title/position of action officer
c) Title/position of individual notifying action officer (if applicable)
d) Time and date action officer was first notified
e) Additional comments

5. Ask questions about procedural knowledge
a) Does your HD have a formal procedure for triaging concerning case reports
b) Is your HD able to record calls for quality assurance purposes
c) Is your HD able to hand a large surge in reporting of concerning cases
d) Could you initiate a 3-way call right now if necessary?
e) Is there a backup action officer on call that could respond to this call?

6. Conclude Call
a) Ask if the action officer has any remaining questions
b) Ensure once again the action officer understands the call was a test
c) Thank the action officer for their time

Training Session 2: Practice and Observation

Knowledge Assessment

1. What should the caller do if they get disconnected from the action officer before he or she is properly debriefed?

2. What should the caller do if they are having trouble getting past the public health agency receptionist or answering service operator?

3. What should the caller do if an action officer is upset by a call?

4. What should the caller do if they reach a dead end phone system?

5. When does debriefing occur for Level 4 tests and how does this differ from Levels 1–3?

6. What should the caller tell a concerned action officer who is worried that the caller are not who they say they are?

7. How long should the caller wait for a callback?

8. What does the caller do if an action officer never calls them back?

9. What does the caller do if they get a respondent who is unable to respond to a Level 3 call?

10. Whom should the caller contact if they have any questions regarding call procedures or have any problems with calls?

Appendix D.
Answers to Knowledge Assessments

<u>Knowledge Assessment 1 Answers</u>

1. What is the purpose of public health disease reporting systems?
Public health disease reporting systems are systems developed by public health agencies to receive case reports from health care workers, usually by telephone. These systems are designed to aid in the early detection of diseases of public health importance and to aid public health agency officials in tracking reportable diseases.

2. How often should public health agencies test their public health disease reporting systems?
The CDC recommends that public health agencies test their public health disease reporting systems at least once annually.

3. What is an "action officer" and what roles and responsibilities does he/she they have?
An action officer is a public health professional whose responsibility is to respond to concerning case reports placed by health care workers to public health disease reporting systems. Action officers can be public health agency directors, epidemiologists, bioterrorism coordinators, doctors, nurses, etc. Action officers should have sufficient training and clinical knowledge to be able to respond appropriately to 80% of all the calls made to a public health agency.

4. What are the three major elements of all tests?
Initiating a call
Reaching an action officer
Debriefing

5. Why is responding to case reports as soon as possible so important?
Responding to case reports quickly and appropriately can reduce the spread of potentially contagious diseases. It also ensures that any questions healthcare workers may have for public health agency officials are answered as soon as possible.

6. What form of communication is the primary means for public health disease reporting systems and why?
The CDC recommends that telephones be used as the primary means for public health disease reporting systems. There are three reasons for this. First telephones allow for a more fluid dialogue of the problem at hand and allow callers reporting concerning cases the ability to ask public health agency officials questions. Second, using telephones reduces the chances that an important case might fall through the cracks (e.g., a fax doesn't get received or noticed immediately, e-mail system errors, etc.). Third, telephones offer a consistent means of communication with public health agencies because all public health agencies across the country have a telephone.

7. What is the maximum amount of time that the CDC recommends for action officers to respond to concerning case reports?
The CDC recommends that all calls to public health agencies regarding concerning cases be responded to in 30 minutes or less.

8. What is a lead-in?
A lead-in is a message that moves a call from a reception desk or answering service to an action officer. It is composed of the caller's name and hospital affiliation, and the request to speak with someone about a patient—a "concerning case." The lead-in never includes any case details.

9. What are the major elements of a proper debriefing?
Clarification that the call is a test that requires no further action
General information about the tests and testing procedures
Contact information for the testing supervisor or coordinator
Questions for respondents

10. Describe ways in which calls that involve the use of a disguise differ from calls that do not involve a disguise.
Calls that involve disguise require callers during call initiation to pretend to be an actual healthcare professional calling about a concerning case.

1. What should the caller do if they get disconnected from the action officer before he or she is properly debriefed?

Callers who get disconnected from an action officer before they are properly debriefed should immediately call the action officer back.

2. What should the caller do if they are having trouble getting past the public health agency receptionist or answering service operator?

Tell the receptionist that the case information is confidential and that you need to speak to whomever in the public health agency is responsible for dealing with cases involving an infectious disease.

3. What should the caller do if an action officer is upset by a call?

If the action officer is upset by the length of time it took them to respond—try to reassure them that there are many places in which a public health disease reporting system can fail and that their response is only one component of that system.

If the action officer is upset by the use of a disguise—explain to them that disguises enhance the realism of a test and help to evaluate public health disease reporting systems in the most realist environment possible.

All calls that involve someone who is upset should also be referred to the testing coordinator.

4. What do the caller do if they reach a dead end phone system?

Record the call as a failure and place the next call according to the call schedule.

5. When does debriefing occur for Level 4 tests and how does this differ from Levels 1–3?

Debriefing for Level 4 calls happens after the caller reaches an action officer and first presents them with information regarding a concerning case that requires their advice. Debriefing for Level 1–3 calls happens immediately after reaching an action officer. Never hang up the phone with an action officer until they have been properly debriefed.

6. What should the caller tell a concerned action officer who is worried that the caller is not who they say they are?

Tell the action officer that they can contact whoever at the public health agency consented for the exercise (usually the public health agency director) directly to verify the authenticity of the test.

7. How long should the caller wait for a callback?

Callers should wait for callbacks for as long as it takes to receive a callback. If the caller will not have access to the telephone line they used to place a call, they should be sure that the telephone has a voicemail or an answering machine that tells respondents that the call is only a test that requires no further action.

8. What should the caller do if an action officer never calls them back?

Record the call as a failure and ensure that after the test at the public health agency has been completed that all public health agency employees are debriefed about the test.

9. What does the caller do if they get a respondent who is unable to respond to a Level 3 call?

Ask the respondent to call an action officer who is able to respond to the call and have that action officer call you back.

10. Whom should callers contact if they have any questions regarding call procedures or have any problems with calls?

Callers should contact their testing coordinator if they have any questions or difficulties during testing.

Appendix E: Testing Template Materials

<u>Lead-in template: Initiating calls that don't involve a disguise</u>

"This is a test of your public health agency's public health disease reporting system. Can you please connect me with the person in this public health agency whose responsibility it would be to respond to a healthcare professional calling about a concerning case involving an infectious disease?"

"This is a test of [name of public health agency]'s public health disease reporting system. The test was authorized by [authorizing individual's name] and is being conducted by [name of testing agency]. Can you please connect me with the person in this public health agency whose responsibility it would be to respond to a healthcare professional calling about a concerning case involving an infectious disease?"

<u>Lead-in template: Initiating calls that involve a disguise</u>

"This is [healthcare professional name and title] calling from [name of local healthcare facility]. I have a concerning case involving an infectious disease that I would like to talk to someone about. Could you please connect me with the appropriate person or have them call me back as soon as possible at [telephone number]?"

"This is Dr. [name]. I am an emergency medicine doctor down here at [local hospital] and I have a case involving what appears to be an infectious disease I would like to talk with whoever handles these sorts of things."

"This is [name]. I am an infectious disease nurse at [local healthcare facility]. I have a patient with some concerning symptoms that I would like to talk about with someone who works in the infectious disease section."

"This is Dr. [name]. I am a geriatrician working at [local nursing home] and I have a patient who has some concerning symptoms that I'd like to talk with someone about. Can you connect me to the appropriate person? The patient appears to have an infectious disease but I am not completely sure."

"This is [name] and I am a school nurse at [local high school]. I have a student here who has some concerning symptoms that I'd like to talk to someone in infectious disease about. Can you connect me to the appropriate person?"

"This message is for [action officer]. My name is [name and title]. I work at [local healthcare facility] and I have a concerning case I would like to discuss with you. It's [date and time]. Could you please call me back as soon as you get this message?"

Debriefing templates

Level 1 Calls

"Thank you for responding to my call. The report you received is part of an exercise being conducted by [name] with the authorization of [name, e.g., director of the public health agency, state public health agency, etc.]. The purpose of this test is to evaluate the public health disease reporting system at your public health agency. The report is not real and requires no further action on your part.

As part of this test, could you please answer the following questions:
- Could you please tell me your job title?
- When did you first receive the information regarding this case?
- What is the job title of the person that contacted you regarding this case?

Thank you again for your participation in this exercise. We ask that you keep this conversation and the exercise in which you just participated confidential. Should you have any questions or concerns and need to contact us, you can contact [name] at [telephone number]."

Level 2 Calls

"Thank you for responding to my call. The report you received is part of an exercise being conducted by [name] with the authorization of [name, e.g., director of the public health agency, state public health agency, etc.]. The purpose of this test is to evaluate the public health disease reporting system at your public health agency. The report is not real and requires no further action on your part.

As part of this test, could you please answer the following questions:
- Could you please tell me your job title?
- When did you first receive the information regarding this case?
- What is the job title of the person that contacted you regarding this case?
- How does your public health agency normally triage case reports?
- What next steps would you take?
- What additional information about this case would you ask for?
- Whom would you routinely notify?

Thank you again for your participation in this exercise."

For tests that involve the use of a disguise, also say: "We ask that you keep this conversation and the exercise to which you just participated confidential. Should you have any questions or concerns and need to contact us, you can contact [name] at [telephone number]."

Level 3 Calls

"Thank you for responding to my call. The report you received is part of an exercise being conducted by [name] with the authorization of [name, e.g., director of the public health agency, state public health agency, etc.]. The purpose of this test is to determine if the appropriate action officer or individual with the authority to respond to the case report within a reasonable time frame (currently, the Centers for Disease Control suggests a public health agency respond to an urgent case report within 30 minutes or initial receipt), has substantive agent and disease knowledge, and understands the appropriate response protocol to a case report. The report is not real and requires no further action on your part.

As part of this test, could you please answer the following questions:

- Could you please tell me your job title?
- When did you first receive the information regarding this case?
- What is the job title of the person that contacted you regarding this case?
- How does your public health agency normally triage case reports?
- What next steps would you take?
- What additional information about this case would you ask for?
- Whom would you routinely notify?

Thank you again for your participation in this exercise. We ask that you keep this conversation and the exercise in which you just participated confidential. Should you have any questions or concerns and need to contact us, you can contact [name] at [telephone number].

Level 4 Calls

Thank you for responding to my call. The report you received is part of an exercise being conducted by [name] with the authorization of [name, e.g., director of the public health agency, state public health agency, etc.]. The purpose of this test is to determine if the appropriate action officer or individual with the authority to respond to the case report within a reasonable time frame (currently, the Centers for Disease Control suggests a public health agency respond to an urgent case report within 30 minutes or initial receipt), has substantive agent and disease knowledge, and understands the appropriate response protocol to a case report. The report is not real and requires no further action on your part.

Just to be sure, do you understand that this is a test, and not a real emergency? Yes/no

As part of this test, could you please answer the following questions:

- Could you please tell me your job title?
- When did you first receive the information regarding this case?
- What is the job title of the person that contacted you regarding this case?

- How does your public health agency normally triage case reports?
- What next steps would you take?
- What additional information about this case would you ask for?
- Whom would you routinely notify?

Before I hang up, I would like to ask you two additional questions:
1) Before I told you this was a test, was it stressful for you to respond to a call regarding a case with the characteristics I've described? [Not at all upsetting/ a little upsetting/very upsetting]
2) Knowing now that you received a 'fake call' as part of the testing procedure, do you find it upsetting that you were misled in order to conduct this test? [Very stressed/a little stressed/not at all stressed]

Note: If stressed: We apologize for stressing you out. We feel the use of a disguise is necessary so that we can understand how public health agencies respond to real emergencies. Was the level of stress you experienced so severe that you think it is problematic to test public health agencies in this way? Y/N

Thank you again for your participation in this exercise. We ask that you keep this conversation and the exercise to which you just participated confidential. Should you have any questions or concerns and need to contact us, you can contact [Name] at [Telephone Number].

Level 3 and 4 case report templates

Case 1: Possible Anthrax

Hi: I'm Dr. [name], an ENT physician at [local healthcare facility]. I'm seeing a really weird case and I wanted to discuss it with you. This is a 19-year-old male student who presented two days ago to the Student Health Service with fever of 100.5 degrees and a sore throat. At that time, it seemed he had unilateral cervical adenopathy and two questionable ulcerations at the base of his tongue that were difficult to visualize. Rapid strep was negative and he was sent home with ibuprofen. Yesterday he developed more difficulty breathing, and he was sent to me. He had two ulcerations at the base of his tongue that looked necrotic. I biopsied them and today they are growing large gram + bacilli. The lab thinks this is consistent with anthrax. I feel silly calling you, but I wanted to see what you thought.

1. Is there any other history? *Not that I know of.*
2. Is there any sexual history? *Heterosexual. Not sexually active.*
3. Is there any travel history? *Not that I know of.*
4. *Where is he now? He's on the ENT service at YYY hospital. I thought we needed to keep an eye on his airway.*
5. How sick is he? *He's mildly febrile and uncomfortable, but vital signs are stable.*

61

6. Are there any other culture results? Have you done blood cultures? *No I haven't. It didn't seem necessary until I just got the culture results. I'm pretty surprised. I've called for an ID consult.*

7. Is he in isolation? *No. Our single rooms are full. Do you think we need to move someone out?*

8. Do you know who else he has been in contact with? *Not really, other than the ED staff and the medical student who examined him.*

9. Are the people involved in his care wearing PPE? *I'm wearing gloves and a surgical mask. Given the gram negatives, we figured this wasn't a problem. But the reason I called you is that I guess this could be anthrax. Do I need to do anything else?*

Case 2: Possible Anthrax

Hi: I'm Dr. [name], an ICU doc at [name of local hospital]. I have a 56-year-old man who has been intubated in our ICU for the last 2 days or so. The story is that he was fine until a few days ago when he presented to the ED after 2 days of fever, malaise, and increasingly drenching night sweats. In the ED he was hypotensive and tachypneic and gave a history of chest pain radiating to his shoulders that was different from his MI pain of 2 days ago. He required intubation shortly thereafter. CXR was consistent showed an unexpectedly wide mediastinum, and bilateral pleural effusions, L>R. An ECHO done in the ED did not show a wall motion abnormality or dissecting aneurism. Sputum gram stain revealed gram-positive bacilli and was begun on broad-spectrum antibiotics. Blood cultures have grown gm+ bacilli, which appear in short encapsulated chains on gram stain. The lab tells me that they look like anthrax. I've never seen anthrax before, so thought I should call you in case.

1. Is there any other history? *No.*
2. What kind of work does he do? *He works at the UPS shipping station.*
3. Any travel history? *No.*
4. Where is he now? *He's in the ICU.*
5. How sick is he? *He's, intubated and sedated. So far his vitals and labs are ok.*
6. Is he in isolation? *No. Our single rooms are full. Do you think we need to move someone out?*
7. Do you know who else he has been in contact with? *Not really, other than the ED staff and the medical student who examined him.*
8. Is there anyone else at his work or in his family who is sick? *I don't know yet.*
9. Are the people involved in his care wearing PPE? *I'm wearing gloves and a surgical mask. The rest of our team put on gowns and masks after we got the call from the lab. Do I need to do anything else?*

Case 3: Possible Botulism

Hi. I'm calling from [name of local hospital]. I'm a medical student from [name of local medical school]. I'm sorry to bother you, but I'm worried that I'm seeing a patient with botulism, and want to know if this could be right. We have a 65-year-old man who was brought to the emergency room after complaining of blurred vision and slurred speech. He has a history of a prior MI and atrial fibrillation, and takes warfarin and a beta blocker. He was generally been feeling well, and played badminton with his grandchildren at a church picnic yesterday. He denies any chest pain, palpitations or headache. In the emergency department, he was alert but his speech was slurred. His visual acuity is 20/40 in both eyes, but his eyelids are drooping (ptosis) bilaterally and his pupils are mildly dilated. His gag reflex is diminished. Sensation, motor strength in his arms and legs, and deep tendon reflexes are intact. While getting an MRI, he aspirated on his secretions, had a respiratory arrest and is now intubated. Over the last few hours he's been getting worse, and now has weakness in his upper extremities. A Tensilon test was negative, as was an MRI. We're now getting ready to do an LP, but I wanted to talk with someone about whether there have been any cases of botulism.

Case 4: Possible Botulism

Hi. I'm Dr. [name] from the ED at [name of local hospital]. I'm seeing a student from [local university] who was brought to the emergency room complaining of double vision. She now has slurred speech and dilated pupils. At first we thought she'd OD'd, but all the toxicology screens are negative. Unfortunately she aspirated her charcoal so we intubated her. The EMS guys say they've had 3 or 4 other runs kind of like this today, with neurologic symptoms that required intubation, so I wanted be sure you knew. Is there something up?

Case 5: Possible Plague

Hi, I'm [name], an infection control nurse at [name of local hospital] in [name of area]. I want to make someone aware of a case I'm worried about.

We have a 42-year-old flight attendant who is hypotensive on a vent in our ICU. The story is that he showed up for work at the airport this morning, and while waiting for his inbound flight, felt flushed. By the time his aircraft was at the gate, he felt feverish and too weak to fly, was thought by some of the other crew to be a bit confused. He was brought to the ED, where he was found to be hypotensive, and tachypneic.

He gave a history of being HIV positive, on meds, and said that his last viral load was low. He became too tachypneic to talk, and was intubated and sedated. His CXR was consistent with ARDS. There are gram-negative bacilli on his sputum gram stain. The attending physician thinks he has an AIDS-associated infection and told me not to worry, but I just got back from a course for ICPs (infection control practitioners) on bioterrorism, and I'm worried this could be something else. Are you seeing other cases like this?

1. Is there any other history? *No.*
2. You said the guy is a flight attendant. Is there any travel history? *We can't get any more history. He works for United Airlines.*
3. Where is he now? *He's in the ICU.*
4. How sick is he? *He's hypotensive on drips, intubated and sedated. So far his labs are ok.*
5. Is he in isolation? *No. Our single rooms are full. Do you think we need to move someone out?*
6. Is there anyone else around to get a history from? *No one has come in yet. He apparently lives in Los Angeles. We've tried calling the home number and the next of kin he listed, but no one has answered yet.*
7. Do you know who else he has been in contact with? *Not really, other than the ED staff and the medical student who examined him.*
8. Are the people involved in his care wearing PPE? *I'm wearing gloves and a surgical mask. Given the gram negatives, we figured this wasn't a problem. But the reason I called you is that I guess this could be plague. Do I need to do anything else?*

Case 6: Possible Smallpox
Hi. My name is [name]. I'm a nurse practitioner at [name of local clinic].

I'm calling because I've seen a couple of strange patients, and I just thought I should check in with you.

Two days ago, I saw a 42-year-old businessman at [hospital] with a fever, headache, and backache. He had been on a recent business trip through Southeast Asia. He wasn't all that ill, so we hydrated him in clinic, and sent of some malaria smears. Today he came back, and was feeling worse. The smears are negative, and on exam, he seems to be getting a rash on his face, arms, and legs. It looks the same all over. He said he hasn't taken any antibiotics or herbal medicines.

The thing that worries me is that yesterday I saw a guy with a similar story and rash, and just now I saw a lady with the same thing. I know this is crazy, but given all the hype about bioterrorism, I'm worried that I could be missing something. Have you heard about other cases like this?

1. Where is he now? *He's here in the emergency department.*
2. How sick is he? *His vital signs are stable, but he looks acutely ill.*
3. Is he in isolation? *Not yet. What kind of isolation do you think he needs?*
4. Can you tell me more about his travel history? *It sounds like he travels a lot. In the last three months he's been all over Southeast Asia. Mostly in cities, but he said he took a short vacation and was in the mountains in Thailand.*
5. Do you know who else he has been in contact with? *Not really, other than the ED staff and the medical student who examined him.*

6. Are you wearing PPE? *I'm wearing gloves. Do I need to do anything else?*
7. I'd like to see him. Can you keep him there? *I'll try, but he says he is planning on leaving tomorrow for another business trip.*
8. Where are the other patients now? *I don't know.*
9. Do you know who they are? *I could probably go back over our clinic logs and figure it out.*

Case 7: Possible Smallpox
Hello: This is Dr. [name] from [name of local clinic].

I have a 21-year-old college student who I was asked to see for fever and rash. She presented two days ago to the Student Health Center with a fever, chills, and headache, and was sent home with Tylenol. Her nasal flu swab was negative [can't use last part if not flu season] The next day she returned with a new rash on her face and arms, but gave a history of taking some of her roommate's trimethoprim-sulfa.

I was asked to see her to determine whether this is a drug rash or chicken pox, and I have to tell you that I'm kind of concerned. First of all, she had a prodrome, and second, all of the lesions on her arms are in the same stage of development.

Have you heard of any other cases like this?

I'm a little worried that this could be smallpox, but it seems kind of unlikely as this would be the first time smallpox was ever reported. What do you think I should do?

1. Where is she now? *She's here in the emergency department.*
2. Is there any travel history? *I don't know. She's a student and I didn't ask.*
3. How sick is she? *Her vital signs are stable, but she looks acutely ill.*
4. Is she in isolation? *Not yet. What kind of isolation do you think she needs?*
5. Do you know whom else she has been in contact with? *Not really, other than the ED staff and the medical student who examined her.*
6. Are you wearing PPE? *I'm wearing gloves. Do I need to do anything else?*
7. I'd like to see her. Can you keep her there? *I'll try, but she's crying and says she just want to go be with her boyfriend. Do you think I should call security? I just asked her to wait, and she says she's going back to her dorm and you can see her there.*

65

Appendix F.
Sample Data Collection Materials

Telephone Information Form (to be completed prior to making calls for all levels)

Performance Criterion	Data	Notes
Single number available for all calls day or night		
Telephone number available through local directory assistance		
Single telephone number well publicized (e.g., same number found in more than one source)		
Total number of telephone numbers at public health agency related to public health disease reporting		

Timeliness of Response Form (to be used with Levels 1–4)

Performance Criterion	Data	Notes
Date and time of call		
Caller's name		
Was the call answered within 5 rings?		
Length of wait time on hold in seconds		
Was the call transferred in 5 rings?		
Was the transfer a *warm transfer*		
Was the call a *dead end* call?		
Length of wait for call back in minutes		
Did you receive the callback in 30 minutes or less?		

Procedural Knowledge Form (to be used with Levels 2–4)

Performance Criterion	Data	Notes
Was the call responded to by an appropriate action officer on first callback or transfer?		
Did the action officer know if their public health agency has a formal triage protocol for concerning case reports? Was the description clear or confusing?		
Did the action officer know whom he or she would contact next?		
Was the action officer aware of whether public health agency has the ability to record calls for quality assurance?		
Did the action officer know about surge capacity for the public health agency's public health disease reporting system?		
Did the action officer know whether or not he or she could initiate a three-way call for concerning case reports?		
Could the action officer establish a three-way call if necessary (e.g., do they know how to do it)?		
Did the action officer know whether or not a backup action officer was available during the time of the call?		
Who is the backup on duty if the action officer is not available?		
How long would it take the backup to respond to the call?		

Content Knowledge Form (to be used with Levels 3 and 4)

Performance Criterion	Data	Notes
Did the action officer ask for the caller's name and contact information?		
Did the action officer determine the disease being discussed in the case report without being told by the caller?		
Did the action officer discuss personal protective equipment with the caller without first being probed?		
Did the action officer ask for more case details after hearing case report?		
What questions did the action officer ask?		
Did the action officer have a clear response plan for moving forward?		
What feedback did the action officer give regarding what to do with the case?		
Did you feel satisfied at the end of the call that the action officer was in control of the situation?		
How long was the call?		

Appendix G.
CDC Performance Criteria for Public Health Disease Reporting Systems Operating 24/7

INTRODUCTION

The performance criteria described here are a product of the *8-City Enhanced Terrorism Surveillance Project*, a CDC initiative focused on strengthening key components of traditional public health surveillance in major metropolitan areas.

The criteria were developed on the basis of findings from site visits to eight major metropolitan areas conducted during February–March 2003 to complete an assessment of promising practices and needs associated with early detection of a terrorist event. This document was subsequently developed as a resource for state and local public health agencies and is intended to represent minimum acceptable criteria. Each public health agency is encouraged to determine the feasibility of implementation and establish a reasonable timeframe, taking into consideration available resources and other competing priorities. If the resources and needs support doing so, public health agencies might also elect to implement more stringent standards of performance.

PERFORMANCE CRITERIA FOR 24/7 REPORTING SYSTEMS:

The performance criteria for each of the 24/7 Reporting Standards are as follows:

Receipt of Initial Report

Standard 1 The telephone should be the primary means for immediate reporting because it is the most direct, rapid, and easy-to-use method for urgent disease reporting of outbreaks or other suspected terrorism threats or public health emergencies. Procedures that can be used by public health agencies fall into three main categories:

> (1a) A physician, laboratory worker, nurse, or other caller telephones the 24/7 number for the public health agency directly. The call is taken by the public health professional on call who accepts the case report; this individual should be capable of handling approximately 80% of the queries received related to infectious disease recognition, diagnosis, and public health management. If further clinical consultation is needed, this health professional arranges a conference call among the caller, himself/herself, and a public health physician (or, if needed, an infectious disease clinician, laboratorian, or other knowledgeable person), or otherwise facilitates the connection between the caller and the resource needed. This system has the advantage of immediate connection of the caller with a public health professional; however, a possible disadvantage exists if this public health professional is unable to directly answer the telephone.

(2) A physician telephones a single 24/7 number set up by the city/state government, or by the public health agency, to handle after-hours calls. The call center staffer conferences in the public health agency professional on call (a warm transfer), who then proceeds as previously described. This system allows for the call center staffer to use a call-down list to locate a public health professional to take the call in situations where the primary on-call staff member is not available, too busy, or unable to be reached. This system also allows the call center staffer to connect incoming calls from physicians to a public health agency on call physician, and other callers to a non-physician public health professional, according to state/local protocol. It also allows the call center staffer to direct the call to an appropriate voice-mail if the call is not urgent.

(3) The third option is similar to the second except that the call-center operator takes the contact information from the calling physician and has the on-call public health professional (or on-call physician) return the call. It has the same advantages as the second procedure.

Performance criteria for Standard 1

All public health agencies should have the ability to receive a report 24/7 via telephone communication with a trained public health professional who is able to handle up to 80% of incoming queries. The trained public health professional should be reachable: (a) directly, (b) via an answering service with immediate ("warm") transfer to the public health professional, or (c) via an answering service with a callback from the public health professional. If the designated public health professional is unavailable, the caller should be able to reach a trained backup public health staff person. The operator or voice mail message should connect with, or inform the caller how to contact, the designated backup staff.

Standard 2 Certain standards should be established to ensure a reliable and rapid means to receive and immediately respond to notifiable diseases and health conditions.

Single telephone number
Components
- Single, well-publicized telephone number (ensure that local directory assistance has this number).
- Triage protocol for incoming calls (see accompanying resource document entitled *24/7 Phone Triage Protocol for Public Health Agencies*).
- Trained professionals to answer the initial call.
- Backup when surge capacity is exceeded [e.g., answering service, voice message (after a maximum number of rings, the caller's telephone number should be recorded for call-back)].
- Public health agency call-down protocol/schedule for 24/7 duty officer

(call-down protocol outlines the names, contact information, and procedures to follow if the primary public health agency respondent is unavailable and a backup must be called).

- Telephone system must have always-on conference call capability.

Performance criteria for Standard 2

Please see the accompanying *24/7 Phone Triage Protocol for Public Health Agencies*, which provides additional guidance for handling incoming calls to 24/7 reporting lines.

Public health agencies should:
1. Implement a single telephone number for 24/7 reports (day and night) for at least acute communicable diseases or acute outbreaks;
2. Provide this single telephone number to directory assistance;
3. Ensure that calls roll over at night/weekend/holiday to on-call public health staff or an answering service;
4. If using an answering service, train answering service staff on the triage protocol for incoming calls to ensure they know the appropriate on-call staff to contact, in addition to when and how to contact them. Each new answering service staff member should be trained before starting to answer calls; all answering service staff should receive refresher training on at least a semiannual basis. A quality-assurance mechanism should be in place for monitoring and evaluating timeliness and quality of handling calls;
    a. Public health staff who answer calls should be trained on triage protocols for incoming calls (contained in a regularly updated on-call manual that also contains key background materials and forms) and know when to contact their supervisors and specialists. Each new public health staff member should be trained before starting to answer calls and all public health staff who handle calls should receive refresher training on at least a semiannual basis. Periodic seminars should be conducted for on-call public health staff to address common on-call topics and acute new issues. The training materials and triage protocol should be available on a restricted access website;
5. Determine the flow of telephone calls if the answerer/line is busy (e.g., transfers to answering machine, keeps ringing, transfers to another number, or caller receives message to stay on line). Ideally, the caller should never get a busy signal. Under conditions of high-volume traffic, the caller should be referred to voice-mail or be placed on hold (with a message stating how many callers are ahead of the caller and an option for the caller to select a voice-mail option).
6. Determine how many rings should occur before the caller is transferred to voice-mail or another person, or receives a message to stay on the line. The call should be transferred within 5 rings;

7. Determine, if the call goes to voice-mail, how many calls can be left on the answering machine (i.e., surge capacity). Where feasible, the answering machine should be able to hold at least 100 three-minute calls;
8. Determine, if a caller is placed on hold, how many callers can remain on the line. Where feasible, the system should have the capacity to hold at least 15 persons on the line;
9. Determine, if a call is transferred to another person or operator, how many others are available. When the maximum number is reached, then a backup system (as noted in the previous item) should be in place;
10. Provide a written list as well as a restricted access website list of those persons who may be called for backup;
11. Keep this backup list up-to-date and make changes as necessary;
12. List at least three persons available for backup and the means to reach them (e.g., pager, home telephone, cellular phone); and
13. Be able to connect at least three people simultaneously on a telephone call. It is recommended that this should be able to be done while in the office and also while out of the office (e.g., home line or cellular phone). This may be accomplished by establishing a conference calling account with a commercial service.

Standard 3 For urgent reports, the time from initial receipt of the call to a response by the public health agency on call physician should not exceed 30 minutes.
Components:
- Primary and backup on-call responders.
- Time limit on callback to triage number to verify receipt.
- Support immediate notification of the state public health agency in accordance with   state/local agreement.

Performance criteria for Standard 3

For recommendations regarding a time limit on the callback to the triage number to verify receipt, please refer to the *24/7 Phone Triage Protocol for Public Health Agencies*.

Public health agencies should ensure that any report of an immediately notifiable illness (including Category A, B, and C agents; occurrence of any unusual disease; and outbreaks of any disease) should be responded to by a public health professional—ideally, a clinically trained public health professional—within 30 minutes of the time the call is made to the public health agency. In addition to the primary on call public health professional, the public health agency should have a minimum of three backup personnel available after normal business hours as part of the 24/7 reporting system. Public health agency staff should document responses to reports or calls in a log book or database. The suspicion or confirmation of any immediately notifiable illness, including category A, B or C agents; unusual disease; and outbreaks of any disease should be reported to the state public health agency, by telephone, within 30 minutes of a local public health professional being notified.

Standard 4 If the telephone system fails, public health agencies must be able to receive urgent reports. Depending on the severity of the situation, a number of alternatives are possible.

- Internet-based reporting (if the provider has a cable or other non-telephone Internet connection, reporting via e-mail or other Internet-based mechanism might be established).
- Cellular phones.
- Satellite phones or radios might be available in critical hospitals.
- Active surveillance (in an emergency, send staff to all or a sample of area hospitals on a daily basis to receive disease reports).

Performance criteria for Standard 4

It is recommended that public health agencies should adopt at least one alternative means for receiving urgent reports in the event of a telephone system failure. Suggested alternative methods include Internet-based reporting with non-telephone Internet connections, cellular phones, on-site radio systems, and satellite phones. States have considered redundant and backup systems as part of their Health Alert Networks (HANs) that might be a resource for local public health agencies in meeting this standard. Information regarding such alternative methods needs to be widely disseminated throughout the area where the primary means of telephone reporting might fail. Active surveillance (manually contacting or even sending staff to visit major hospitals on a daily basis to receive disease reports) is recommended as a tertiary method of receiving disease reports.

Education and Awareness

Standard 5 Information on disease reporting requirements (when, what, who, where, and why to report) should be communicated to clinicians and laboratorians and should include the following:

- Clear public health contact information.
- Encouragement to report pre-diagnoses and suspicions.
- Education regarding reasons to report.
- Regular feedback from the public health agency to providers that reports have been received and how the information is being used.
- Education regarding what diagnoses (suspected or confirmed) and laboratory findings are immediately reportable.

Performance criteria for Standard 5

These performance criteria relate to the content of education and awareness materials.

It is recommended that public health agencies should review informational materials for their 24/7 reporting systems, initially and on an annual basis thereafter. Such review should document the existence of non-ambiguous, accurate contact information. Evidence should exist that clinicians, laboratories, and other healthcare professionals are explicitly asked to report to and consult with the public health agency even if they merely suspect the presence of a Category A, B, or C agent; occurrence of any unusual disease; or outbreaks of any disease. Any changes in state reporting requirements should also be considered during this review. All informational materials to promote 24/7 reporting should illustrate the reasons why early and consistent reporting is important to safeguard public health. Information regarding 24/7 reporting should specify that the telephone is the most appropriate means for immediate reporting both during and after business hours. The content of education and awareness materials should include a written list of all notifiable diseases with brief reports to the clinical community and any other group submitting notifiable-disease reports, describing key examples of reported cases of notifiable diseases and summarizing actions taken.

Standard 6 Multiple outreach mechanisms should be used to disseminate educational information, including

- Partnerships with local authorities for clinicians and professional societies.
- Personal office visits.
- Internet, mail, meeting presentations, or stickers.
- National campaigns using alternative outreach mechanisms.
- Speakers' bureaus and health-care provider focus groups.

Performance criteria for Standard 6

These performance criteria relate to outreach mechanisms for education and awareness materials.

Public health agencies should integrate at least two of the following methods of disseminating information into their routine education and awareness programs through use of working partnerships between local authorities and professional societies to disseminate information to the societies' members: marketing devices such as calendars, stickers, and magnets; physician office visits; meeting presentations; the Internet; and mailings. If public health agency staff cannot make personal office visits to physicians, this could be accomplished through partnerships with pharmaceutical company representatives or through laboratory chains in their contact with physician offices. (State public health agencies might also be able to provide support for local outreach efforts and might already have spent time and resources to establish communications and outreach mechanisms that could be used.)

Standard 7 The target audience for education and awareness materials should be defined [e.g., infection control practitioners (ICPs), clinicians (both hospital and office based), labs, school nurses, occupational health offices, child care providers, food establishments, nursing homes, veterinarians and animal handlers, correctional health facilities, and healthcare facilities (hospitals, long-term care, urgent care, and health-plan directors)].

Performance criteria for Standard 7

These performance criteria relate to who is to receive education and awareness materials.

Public health agencies should review and define their current and potential target audiences for education and awareness on 24/7 reporting, initially and on an annual basis thereafter. Audiences should be prioritized based upon their likelihood of seeing patients with diseases resulting from a terrorism event, or the laboratory specimens from such patients (both clinical and forensic laboratories), so that education and awareness activities are addressed to the highest priority audiences first. Consideration may be given to more specific identification of clinicians who might serve as sentinel physicians to model desired reporting behavior. Rather than requiring that any specific groups be included as a target audience, the proposed performance criteria emphasize that the approach to defining the target audience be conducted in a planned and systematic manner as opposed to an ad hoc manner.

Standard 8 Disease reporting requirements should reach licensed physicians, or subsets delineated by specialty or practice types, and laboratories on at least an annual basis.

Performance criteria for Standard 8

These performance criteria relate to penetration and frequency of distribution for education and awareness materials.

For public health agencies that have not distributed information regarding disease reporting requirements to all licensed physicians within their jurisdictions in the last year, such information should be disseminated. Public health agencies should also review, and if necessary revise, their disease reporting requirements each year and send this information to all licensed physicians on an annual basis. The penetration of currently practicing licensed physicians and laboratories reached should be at least 90% and 95%, respectively.

In the event of a change in reporting requirements between the time of the annual review and dissemination of reporting requirements, an alert to all licensed physicians should be sent within 30 days of the change in reporting requirements. If changes occur in reporting requirements for specific subsets (e.g., laboratories), it is recommended that public health agencies should have the capability to identify and send the changes to these specific subsets within 30 days of the change in reporting requirements. The penetration of currently practicing licensed physicians and laboratories reached should be at least 90% and 95%, respectively.

In addition to the annual dissemination of disease reporting requirements and alerting when changes have occurred in disease reporting requirements, public health agencies should post the information regarding disease reporting requirements on their Internet sites.

Standard 9 The process by which cases of marker diseases of immediate public health importance (e.g., meningococcal meningitis, SARS, rabies, botulism) are reported is a reasonable proxy for how cases due to terrorism agents would be reported in a given jurisdiction. Examples of ways in which this could be measured include the following:

- What percentage of those cases that should come through the 24/7 reporting system actually do (as compared to paper or fax reporting)?
- What percentage of calls come in for consultation before a diagnosis is made?

Performance criteria for Standard 9

These performance criteria relate to evaluation of both the 24/7 reporting system and education and awareness materials.

Evaluation of the 24/7 reporting system

- It is recommended that a plan for a terrorism-oriented evaluation of the 24/7 reporting system be developed [MMWR 1999;48(RR-11)]. The plan should include the following:

  1. Identification of stakeholders who will implement the evaluation, including staff who operate the system, representatives of outside healthcare providers who use the system, and other interested persons (e.g., internal and external professional staff).
  2. Description of the 24/7 reporting system, including the organizational structure and resources used to operate it.
  3. A list of marker diseases that serve as a proxy for how cases caused by terrorism agents would be reported. Potential marker diseases are listed in the standard.
  4. A list of questions to be answered through the evaluation of the marker diseases, a description of data and information required to answer each of the questions, and an indication of how the data and/or information will be gathered. Potential questions include those listed in the standard. Proposed performance criteria for the questions in the standard are as follows: (a) at least 90% of cases were identified through the 24/7 reporting system; and (b) for the marker diseases, Category A, B, and C agents that the public health agency has determined should be immediately reported, and any other unusual diseases or outbreaks, > 80% of calls should come in for consultation relative to suspicion of disease before diagnosis.

5. Description and results of any formal system testing related to this evaluation (see Standards 10 and 11).
6. Description of how the findings from the evaluation will be disseminated and used (i.e., who will receive conclusions and recommendations and how will the recommendations be acted upon).
7. A schedule for gathering, analyzing, and interpreting data and information; making conclusions and forming recommendations; and disseminating findings from the evaluation.

- As resources permit, public health agencies should implement this evaluation and disseminate conclusions and recommendations. This evaluation should be done as often as needed or at least every 2 years.

Evaluation of education and awareness materials

- To assess the degree of penetration of information regarding reporting requirements, and to identify possible problems in the methods of dissemination, a rapid and simple survey should be conducted on an annual basis, 30 days after the dissemination of information regarding reporting requirements, to subsets of licensed physicians to determine if they have recalled receiving the reporting requirements, whether or not they have read the reporting requirements, and what they consider to be the best communication channel to use for future information dissemination (mail, fax, and/or e-mail). Such a survey in itself would also help to raise awareness of the reporting requirements. Each public health agency should formally review the results of such an annual survey and take appropriate corrective actions to solve problems identified. Alternate methods of information dissemination (e.g., fax and e-mail in addition to regular mail) should be considered as appropriate.

Testing of 24/7 Reporting System

Standard 10 Regular, formal, unannounced standardized system testing (i.e., not relying on daily use as a test mechanism) should be implemented to assess the following components:
- Existence/use of standard protocols
- Whether the call connects
- Who answers the call
- How quickly the caller reaches an action officer
- How quickly consultation is initiated
- Review of the call response (recording or listening in)
- Backup and surge capacity.

Standard 11 Testing should be conducted at least annually

A protocol for formal testing of the 24/7 reporting system should be developed and implemented on at least an annual basis. The protocol should cover the following:

1. Assignment and responsibilities of the system and staff who will conduct the testing.
2. Performance criteria include: (a) the test being unannounced except to the health officer and person conducting the test; (b) the call being connected to an actual person; (c) the caller being connected to the on call or designated backup person within 30 minutes; (d) the caller reaching a clinically trained public health professional within 30 minutes; (e) a three-way conference with a clinical specialist being arranged within an additional 30 minutes, if needed; (f) the telephone call being recorded for training and quality control purposes; (g) the system of reporting being tested both during and after normal business hours.
3. The expected frequency of testing should be at least annually.
4. A description of how and to whom the findings from the testing will be disseminated and how the findings are likely to be acted upon.

The first test under this protocol should be conducted as soon as possible and its findings disseminated to the health officer and all staff involved in the 24/7 alerting system.

Appendix H.
Frequently Asked Questions

Q. Who developed the tests?
A. The RAND Corporation developed and tested these proficiency tests in 2004 under contact from the U.S. Department of Health and Human Services.

Q. How were the tests developed?
A. The tests were initially developed using guidelines developed by the CDC in 2003. They were beta tested at 20 state and local public health agencies across the country from April 2004 until September 2004.

Q. Why does the manual focus on telephone calls as the means for public health disease reporting rather than other modes of communication such as faxes or e-mails?
A. The CDC recommends that telephones be used as the primary means for immediate reporting because they are the most direct, rapid, and easy-to-use method for urgent disease reporting of outbreaks, suspected terrorism threats, or public health emergencies.

Q. How often should public health agencies test their public health disease reporting systems?
A. The CDC recommends that public health agencies test their public health disease reporting systems at least annually.

Q. How long is the typical test of one public health agency?
A. The typical test approximately 1 month to complete.

Q. How many staff members are required to conduct a typical test on one public health agency?
A. A typical test involves 1–3 callers working on average 5 hours a week of testing each. Tests on more than one public health agency can be conducted by the same testing agency; however, multiple tests will require more staff time.

Q. How many calls are required in a typical test?
A. A typical test of one public health agency involves 10 calls.

Q. What is the advantage of Level 4 tests—which may upset staff?
A. First, real emergencies are stressful. Staff members are better able to handle high-stress situations if they have practiced beforehand. Second, most people—even if initially upset—recognize that if a capability is important enough to be tested, it is an important part of their job. The test itself conveys the message that good stress management skills are vital to the department.

Q. Why do callers disguise themselves in some tests?
A. The goal of the tests is to evaluate public health disease reporting systems in an environment that is as realistic as possible. Respondents who know they are participating in a test may respond differently to the test call than they would to a real call. Disguises are used to make the test as realistic as possible.

Q. Should public health agencies self-test or have the tests done by an outside agency?
A. Self-testing provides challenges to individuals in charge or developing a test because it is more difficult to keep the test a secret. Self-testing, however, can often be accomplished more quickly and efficiently than testing from an outside agency.

Q. Why are call schedules necessary?
A. Call schedules are important for two reasons. First, they ensure that public health agencies participating in a test receive calls at different days and times during the week. Second, they ensure that callers know when to place calls.

Q. How many calls does a typical test involve?
A. A typical test involves approximately 10 calls.

Q: Should callers take notes throughout the call?
A: Yes, callers should take notes during and immediately after the call.

Q. May callers take notes on a keyboard or PDA?
A. Only if the keyboard is silent (keyboard clicks lead to immediate detection and tend to disconcert callers).

Q: Callers are still uncomfortable making Level 4 calls, even after practicing. Any advice?
A: Schedule additional practice sessions. Have callers begin with Level 3 calls and gain experience before placing a Level 4 call.

Q: What if I get disconnected when I am making a call?
A: If you are disconnected, it is imperative that you call the action officer back immediately, especially in the event of a Level 4 phone call that has been disconnected before the test is revealed. All possible action should be taken to reconnect with the action officer, even if it is necessary to inform other public health agency staff of the test. When you have reached the action officer, immediately inform him/her of the test. If the action officer has notified other public health professionals of the case, work with the action officer to inform everyone that this is only a test. In addition, the individual(s) supervising the test administration should be informed as soon as possible if this situation occurs.

Q: What if the action officer is upset?
A: The action officer may be upset when the call is revealed to be a test, particularly under the stressful conditions of a Level 4 phone call. If the action officer is extremely upset, apologize for any inconvenience. Tell him or her that the testing coordinator will

call them back to discuss their concerns. Contact the testing coordinator and have them contact the respondent.

Q: What if the action officer questions whether the caller is authorized to conduct the test?
A: Inform the action officer of the testing supervisor that authorized this test. If the action officer is still concerned about answering the test questions, provide them with the contact information for the testing supervisor.

Q: What if the action officer asks how she performed/if she passed?
A: Inform the action officer that her response is only part of the response of the entire public health disease reporting system at the public health agency. It is not recommended that you explicitly judge the performance of the action officer during the debriefing. If necessary, provide the action officer with a summary of the key evaluation points.

Q: How do I know when to debrief during a Level 4 call?
A: The question of when to end Level 4 and debrief is a matter for individual judgment. The use of a disguise should end if all useful information has been extracted or the call is not going well (for example, if the action officer is becoming too stressed to handle the call).

Q: Should callers debrief action officers that have been reached already in the past?
A: Yes. Everyone should be debriefed, even those who receive more than one call.

Q: What if the action officer is aware of the test from others?
A: Even if the action officer is aware of the test from colleagues, the action officer must be fully debriefed.

Q: What if I have not reached the action officer but have started a case description during a Level 4 test?
A: Immediately inform the respondent that this is a test. Inform the respondent of the purpose of and authorization for the test, and ask the respondent not to discuss the test with colleagues. Then, ask the respondent to forward you to the appropriate action officer, but do not inform the action officer of the test immediately. Conduct the test and debriefing.

Q. What should I do if my call is disconnected while I am talking with an action officer?
A. If the call is disconnected prior to or during debriefing, you must regain contact with the individual immediately, by calling the public health agency number again and asking to be transferred to the individual with whom you were just speaking, by calling the action officer directly (if you have the contact information), or, if absolutely necessary, contacting the public health agency director and informing him/her of the situation.

Q. What if the initial public health agency operator needs more information to triage the call to the appropriate action officer?

A. A number of public health agencies have separate sections dealing with STDs, HIV/AIDS, and TB. Use your best judgment in supplying additional information. For instance, you could indicate that your "concerning case" does not appear to be any of the aforementioned. Lead-ins should be vague. Tell the operator that the case information is confidential and ask to be connected with someone in the infectious disease section.

Q: What is the relative importance of the various performance criteria?
A: Each criterion sequentially builds on prior criteria—first it must be possible to find the telephone number, then one must be able to reach a health professional, etc. In this sense, the early criteria are the most fundamental. But all criteria are very important.

Q: How many calls to a public health agency are required before the evaluation?
A: A good rule of thumb is to make at least four calls; as many as seven calls may be necessary if the department will be tested in several different levels.

Q: How quickly should evaluations be performed?
A: It is best to write the evaluation as soon as possible (e.g., within one week) after the call has been completed.

Q: How much flexibility do I have to ask questions, etc., on a call?
A: Conversations with health staff are intended to be relatively open-ended. You may wish to pursue a particular point more fully on some calls than others. When calls and conversations take interesting turns that shed additional light on the department's capacities, don't forget to take detailed notes describing what happened.

Q: How much testing is too much testing?

A: Testing should always be balanced and should not overtax public health agency staff. The goal is to ensure the system is functioning, not to exhaust staff. Public health agencies that have major changes in staffing or the structure of their public health disease reporting system may choose to test their system several times in one year until the system is moving smoothly again. Public health agencies with well-established public health disease reporting systems may choose to evaluate the system only once a year.

Q: Our public health disease reporting system works well. Why should we allocate valuable staff time to test it regularly?
A: The only way to ensure that your public health agency's public health disease reporting system is working is to test it regularly. Many public health agencies that felt they had a well functioning public health disease reporting system found gaps in their system by using the tests outlined in this manual.

Q: The staff in my public health agency resent being tested—what steps can I take alleviate this?
A: Tell staff that the monitoring of performance is now very commonplace in businesses across the country. Emphasize to staff the importance of a well functioning public health disease reporting system. The tests are not designed to evaluate individuals but instead to

evaluate systems. These systems can break down in many places and it is rarely one individual's fault that the system breaks down.

Q: Should I record some calls to use for training and to ensure quality?
A: It is a good idea to set up a system to record a random number of calls to use for training and quality assurance. If this approach is taken, federal law requires that all callers be informed that calls can be recorded for quality assurance purposes.

Appendix I.
Sample After-Action Report

[Date]

[Public health agency Name]

Dear [Public health agency Director]

We tested your public health agency's disease reporting system from [date] until [date], placing [number] calls at various times of day and night, on weekdays as well as weekends.

In this report we summarize your public health agency's performance using four criteria created by the CDC for public health disease reporting systems[6]:

- Was there a phone number available from local directory assistance?

- Was there a single number available for all calls, day or night?

- Could callers reach a public health agency staff member with clinical knowledge *(an action officer)* within 30 minutes, and what percentage of calls received a response in 30 minutes or less?

- Did calls result in immediate connection *(warm transfer)* to an action officer?

[Other criteria can be added to this list and the results from those criteria can be added to the after-action report]

Your public health agency's phone number was [available/not available] from local directory assistance and there [was or was not] one single number for all calls. The longest response time was [number] minutes, [percent] of all calls received a response within 30 minutes, and [percent] were warm transfers. Table 1 contains your public health agency's raw data.

Table 1. Raw data for calls

Call #	Response Time (minutes)	Time of Day	Weekend	Warm Transfer?
1				
2				
3				
4				
5				

---

[6] http://www.cdc.gov/epo/dphsi/files/Performance_Criteria_Public_Health_Disease_Reporting_Systems.doc.

References

Buehler JW, Hopkins RS, Overhage JM, Sosin DM, Tong V. Framework for Evaluating Public Health Surveillance Systems for Early Detection of Outbreaks. MMWR 53(RR05);1–11, 2004.

Centers for Disease Control and Prevention. Guidelines for Evaluating Surveillance Systems. MMWR 37:1–18, 1988.

Centers for Disease Control and Prevention. Updated Guidelines for Evaluating Public Health Surveillance Systems: Recommendations from the Guidelines Working Group. MMWR 50:1–35, 2001.

Centers for Disease Control and Infection. Performance Criteria for Public Health Disease Reporting Systems Operating Twenty-four Hours per Day, Seven Days per Week (24/7); 2003. Available at: http://www.cdc.gov/epo/dphsi/8city.htm

Henderson JM. Testimony before the Subcommittee on Emergency Preparedness and Response, Select Committee on Homeland Security, United States House of Representatives. September 24, 2003. Available at: http://www.hhs.gov/asl/testify/t030924.html

Jajosky RA, Groseclose SL. Evaluation of Reporting Timeliness of Public Health Surveillance Systems for Infectious Diseases. BMC Public Health 4:29, 2004.